INCIDENTAL
FINDINGS

INCIDENTAL FINDINGS

Lessons from My Patients
in the Art of Medicine

DANIELLE OFRI

BEACON PRESS
BOSTON

BEACON PRESS
25 Beacon Street
Boston, Massachusetts 02108-2892
www.beacon.org

Beacon Press books
are published under the auspices of
the Unitarian Universalist Association of Congregations.

Printed in the United States of America

08 07 06 05 8 7 6 5 4 3 2 1

This book is printed on acid-free paper that meets
the uncoated paper ANSI/NISO specifications
for permanence as revised in 1992.

Text design by Bob Kosturko
Composition by Wilsted & Taylor Publishing Services

LIBRARY OF CONGRESS CATALOGING-IN-PUBLICATION DATA

Ofri, Danielle.
  Incidental findings : lessons from my patients in the art of medicine / Danielle Ofri.
    p. ; cm.
  ISBN 0-8070-7266-4 (cloth : alk. paper)
  1. Physicians—Anecdotes. 2. Medicine—Anecdotes. 3. Physician and patient—
Anecdotes.
  [DNLM: 1. Physician-Patient Relations—Personal Narratives. 2. Patients—
psychology—Personal Narratives. 3. Physicians—psychology—Personal
Narratives. W 62 O33i 2004] I. Title.

R705.O38 2004
  610.69'6—dc22   2004021445

The names and many identifying characteristics of patients mentioned in this work
have been changed to protect their identities.

FOR MY PATIENTS

FOR NAAVA AND NOAH

CONTENTS

INCIDENTAL F*i*NDINGS

I HAVE AN MD. I HAVE A PH.D. I'm on the faculty of NYU School of Medicine as an attending physician in the department of medicine. And with all of these qualifications, I am lost. It is 8:30 A.M., and I am on my way to get an amniocentesis and ultrasound for my first pregnancy. *Suite 9V* is what I remember seeing on my calendar this morning, and my husband trusts me because, after all, I am a faculty member here. But this is the new building of NYU private practices, and I normally work at Bellevue Hospital, down the block.

We've finally made it to Suite 9V, but the door says OTOLARYN-GOLOGY.

Otolaryngology? Something is wrong here. I scan up and down the long hallway of gray industrial carpeting. The smell of new paint sours the back of my throat as I hunt for landmarks in what should be familiar territory. There's an office labeled ENDOCRI-NOLOGY and another labeled UROLOGY. How could it not be here? I swear that *9V* was written in my calendar, and I *never* forget details like that. I'm an internist, and remembering details is my stock-in-trade.

This place gives me metallic shivers—it feels more like an office building than a hospital. There doesn't seem to be any hint of humanity or healing in the starkly generic layout. I am lost in my own hospital.

My husband waits for me to decide which way to go next—after all, this is my hospital. My sense of order and organization is feeling wobbly. I know this shouldn't be such a big deal, but I'm annoyed that the room wasn't where I expected it to be and that there aren't any signs to point us in the right direction. My normally assertive doctor stride has given way to more tentative steps as I peer down this corridor and that, squinting for a sign to guide us.

I spy PEDIATRIC CARDIOLOGY. Well that's a start—at least it's about kids. A somber couple is sitting in the small waiting area that is festooned with cheery depictions of elephants and puppies in eye-twitching primary colors.

In a whisper, I ask the receptionist where amnios are done.

"You looking to do an amnio or a cardiac sonogram?" she bellows with operatic resonance.

I can barely muster up enough voice for a reply.

She turns from me. "Sylvia," she hollers out to her colleague at the copier. "Hey Sylvia, we don't do amnios here, do we?" I wince and try to calm my breathing. "Sorry, miss, we only do pediatric sonograms." Fine, but do you know where they do amnios? She shrugs and picks a fleck of dust from under a spiky fingernail. "Try the tenth floor."

My husband and I head for the stairs instead of the elevator. We are starting to run late and I hate—*hate*—being late. The stairwell is painted gray. Why is everything gray? The stairs must have been recently painted, or maybe there's just no ventilation, because the acrid paint smell is intensified. I feel the turpentine vapors invading my lungs as we pant our way up the stairs. This can't be good for me. This can't be good for the baby; I know there's horrible stuff in paint. Could thirty-seven seconds in this hermetically sealed chamber be enough for those chemicals to inflict genetic damage on a fetus? I gulp for fresh—fresh?—air when we push the emergency exit door that threatens to, but luckily doesn't, sound an alarm.

Together we march purposefully down the corridor, determined to find what we are looking for. Then it dawns on me: I don't even *know* what I am looking for. Is it Radiology? Or Obstetrics? Or Genetics? How will I know when I'm there if I don't know what I'm looking for?

Up and down the hallway we traipse and my legs begin tingling in odd places. CARDIOTHORACIC SURGERY. GASTROENTEROLOGY. PULMONOLOGY. The signs are suspended from the ceiling so we have to stagger along with our heads cocked backwards like tourists from Des Moines in Times Square, oblivious to the horizon and all events planar. DERMATOLOGY. NONINVASIVE CARDIOLOGY. VASCULAR SURGERY. Fluorescent light fixtures alternate with the signs. My pupils are assaulted by the direct attack of the lights and I feel the beginnings of vertigo. I lower my eyes from the ceiling and start focusing on the doorways. They are monotonous gray doors with black lettering. The offices are all identical and their bland uniformity is starting to melt into a surreal postmodern moonscape.

Where is the damn room and why isn't there anyone to help us? It is already 8:45, and my stomach is tightening as I realize that we are making my doctor wait. I hate it when my own patients arrive late and have sworn never to be late myself.

We try the eleventh floor. Same carpeting, same doorways, same offices. The gray is making me nauseated. I will never decorate any room of mine in gray. My child will never wear gray. I will dye my hair black or green or orange or anything before it goes completely gray, though time is already running out on that one. I spot a familiar name on a door, a gynecologist on the medical school faculty with whom I've consulted once or twice. My heart jumps an extra beat. The familiarity of a name, any name, a gynecologist no less, makes me exhale balloons of tension. I burst in and am surprised that my voice won't come so easily. Amnio, I pant. Where's amnio?

"Are you a patient of Dr. Levine's?" the receptionist asks politely and all too slowly. No, I say, but I'm getting an amnio and I don't know where to go.

"Well, it all depends," she says, straightening the papers on her desk. "Some doctors like to use the ultrasound suite, some prefer the high-risk OB suite, some do it in their own office. Which does your doctor prefer?"

I stare blankly at her manicured nails and efficiently organized desk with the pink message pads and insurance forms lying at crisp right angles to each other. My mind is melting and I can't put two rational words in sequence. I have no idea what my doctor's personal preference for amniocentesis is and can't even begin to guess.

"Try 7V," she says, placing the tip of her pen thoughtfully against her lower lip. "That's high-risk OB. Are you high-risk?"

High-risk? My eyes fly about the room, flitting desperately from the upbeat David Hockney print to the moralizing breast-feeding poster from La Leche League. Am I high-risk? As a doctor, I know that "advanced maternal age" is considered high-risk, but as a patient, I am suddenly panicked. High-risk? I grab for my husband's hand.

Back in the hallway, now rushing for the stairs, I am suddenly overcome. Tears begin to flow uncontrollably. I am lost, so deeply lost in my fears and this monolithic labyrinth. Where am I supposed to be? What is going to happen to me? My husband is comforting. We'll find it, he reassures me. I feel so silly, bawling because I can't find a stupid room, in my very own hospital no less. It's not as though I'm delivering bad news to a patient, or even getting bad news myself…it's just a goddamned room. But I'm crying and can't seem to stop. What if one of my medical students walks by? The clock is ticking: I'm late, I'm lost, and someone's about to stick a huge needle into my belly. And now I'm high-risk.

My husband leads me into the elevator. Two doctors enter on the next floor. Their white coats are crisp and *Attending Physician* is tidily embroidered over the left pocket of each one. It's the same coat I wear when I'm seeing patients. The same coat that identifies me as a faculty member, as a senior physician, as someone in charge of the well-being of patients and the training of students and young doctors. Their white coats only emphasize how wide the gulf is right now, how distant I feel from my former confident self. I turn my reddened eyes away, hoping they won't recognize me in my civilian garb.

I don't know these doctors personally, but if I were in my white coat, we'd give each other a polite nod, tacitly acknowledging each other as members of the same order. But apparently in my ordinary clothes and tear-stained face, the physician in me is not recognizable. In fact, they don't seem to register my presence at all; I am barely a blip on their radar.

<hr/>

Down another gray hall and there it is. Suite 7V. PERINATAL DIAGNOSTIC UNIT—I never would have guessed that name. My insides shudder at this vision of Mecca, and my legs weaken with relief. We have arrived.

I stagger into the room, or at least I feel like I'm staggering. It has only been twenty-five minutes of wandering the halls but each minute has made me feel worse. The tingling has spread throughout my body and I feel lightheaded. I numbly remove my clothes and change into the stiff, skimpy gown in the subzero room. My doctor bustles in with a cheery hello and starts washing up at the sink. Apparently she's running late too, but that's par for the course for doctors; my own lateness isn't even noticed.

I eye the eerily familiar preparatory rituals of the doctor donning sterile gloves and then swabbing the patient's skin with iodine in ever-widening circles of dark amber, except that the patient is me, and I never realized how frigidly wet the iodine feels on tender, exposed skin. The nurse opens the needle packet for my doctor. I recognize the needle and can identify its length and width just by the color of the packaging. I've stuck that very same needle into many patients—into their spinal canals, their bone marrows, their jugular veins, their lung cavities, and even their bellies. I've plunged in that needle confidently and without flinching, more times than I can count. But this is the first time I've ever faced the business end of the needle. It is metallically menacing, like medieval armor, and far larger than I ever recalled its being.

The doctor presses it into my browned and cleaned belly and it's more than "just a little pinch and a tiny bit of pressure," as she had casually warned me. The shiny lancet sinks deeper and deeper into my insides and there is a sensation I cannot describe. It is pain, yes, but even more, it is violation. It is a violation of my heretofore never penetrated belly. With the luck of good health, I have never been cut open or stitched or instrumented in any way. I have never been a patient in a hospital. Other than a bout of chicken pox as a medical student, I've never even been sick before. And now there is a cold metal object careening its way into my body until the entire impossible length of it has disappeared within.

My doctor has been pushing the needle assertively through the layers of my body, assured by the simultaneous ultrasound that she's not stabbing my kid. I suddenly lose faith in technology and can't believe that the fuzzy images on the ultrasound screen are enough to prevent the impalement of my baby.

All of a sudden, yellow fluid bursts into the syringe attached to the needle—innards of me escaping unnaturally to the outside world. It all seems so backward and inside out. Metal needles that are usually perched calmly on shelves in sterile packages are now deep inside me. My fluids that are supposed to be tucked safely within me are sitting naked and exposed in polypropylene syringes. All of this trustingly based on a technology that suddenly strikes me as the height of shamanism. It's no better than cloves and incantations. It's a wild leap of faith that is flabbergasting in its irrationality. What could I possibly have been thinking when I consented to this?

I close my eyes and pray for the world to right itself.

With a quick snap, the needle is plucked from my belly. The wound is compressed, test tubes capped, needles discarded, gloves snapped off. My doctor packs up her things, gives me a friendly pat on the shoulder, and is off to her next patient before I can even register what I am doing here, much less what post-needle-impalement etiquette should be.

My husband and I are left with the ultrasound technician, who will now do a detailed sonogram of our baby. Exhausted, I let myself go under the technician's confident hands as she skates her probe over my belly, now awash in gobs of bluish jelly. I open my eyes, blink a few times as I adjust to the planet I have landed on, and then with an epiphany that is almost biblical in its intensity, I am suddenly *thrilled* to be a patient.

There it is...that's our baby up on the screen. Our baby!

Comfortably oblivious to our cries of amazement, it sedately shows off its noble profile, displaying its regal toes and cerebellum and contracting ventricles of the heart. And when it's bored with that and us, it rolls over insouciantly to find a more attractive position in its cocoon. With a flick of its delicate upturned nose, it has erased all traumas of the morning. I am no longer lost. I am anchored in this world, as I have never been before. I forgive everything and anything and anyone.

Medicine is a miracle and I am grateful to be its supplicant.

The dreamy sonogram ends and the goose bumps on my skin have begun to recede. The attending radiologist pokes his head in the door just as I am scraping off the last of the sticky jelly. My husband and I are still marveling over the miracles we have just witnessed. The radiologist has already ascertained that I am a doctor and fellow faculty member. "Just one thing," he says, leaning his torso into the room, "the umbilical cord is missing one artery, but it's probably an incidental finding. The literature says that twenty percent can have chromosomal abnormalities, but you've already done the amnio to check for that, and twenty percent can have growth retardation, but we'll be able to check that with another ultrasound in three weeks, so it's probably a normal anatomical variant." His head retreats into the hallway.

A missing what?

Which artery? An important one? Come back here.

I struggle to recall the anatomy of the umbilical cord. I know there is something unique and unbalanced about its structure: is it two arteries and one vein, or two veins and one artery?

Aren't *all* arteries important?

The radiologist pulls himself back into our room at our beseeching cries. "The literature is old," he says with a shrug and a knowing smile to me, a fellow faculty member. "No prospective, randomized clinical trials. You'll know the amnio results in two weeks and we'll do another sono a week later. Nothing to worry about." Out he goes.

My nonmedical husband is fumbling with the idea of missing arteries and I'm trying to unravel memories of embryology lectures from twenty years ago. We grab hands instinctively and the technician takes pity on us. "Between you and me," she says, "I've seen tons of these missing-artery things; it's always nothing. And we do lots of high-risk pregnancies here."

High-risk—that awful word again.

"Many abnormal babies have missing arteries," she says, "but for most missing arteries the babies are normal. Get it?"

I think I do. Maybe. I know that technicians are not supposed to give out any medical information, so I am extra grateful for her words.

We walk out into the sunlight, stepping gingerly since I'm a little sore. But I'm more shaken than sore. I reflect back on how discombobulated I'd become from the simple act of getting lost this morning. How many patients do I send for procedures, many of whom have little education or command of English? How many have wandered the hallways, holding up their referral forms to strangers, hoping someone will have the knowledge and the patience to help them out? How many of my patients give up in frustration and simply go home? I'd never thought about how hard it could be just to *get* there.

And how do we convey mildly bad news? We obviously try to be careful about the big bad news—cancer, HIV, Alzheimer's disease—with sensitive, empathic discussions. But what about the incidental findings—the bit of gastritis seen during an endoscopy, the benign calcification noted on a mammogram, the simple ovarian cyst picked up on a sonogram. For us in the medical profession, these are small potatoes, hardly worth much thought given the more serious issues we must face with our sicker patients. But as I learned today, there is no such thing as incidental to a patient.

Nothing is incidental. The location of the room is not incidental. The "normal anatomical variant" is not incidental. The "little pinch and a tiny bit of pressure" is not incidental. The frigid room and skimpy gowns are not incidental. I want to announce it to the receptionists and the radiologist and the obstetrician and the gray-brained designers of this infernal building. "I am not incidental!" I want to enunciate every syllable. I want it to echo down the sterile carpeted corridors.

I am *not* incidental.

But I am now wiser.

<hr/>

Medical school and residency training had been a long journey, one thankfully completed. But now I was embarking on a new journey toward parenthood. It was a bit like planning a trip to Neptune. Having never been there, and not able to envision it, I didn't know what the weather would be like, what language would be spoken, what the local customs would be. What should I pack? How should I prepare? What should I expect?

I didn't have any answers for these questions but could only go forward on this journey, consigned to figuring it out as I went along. This would also evolve into a path toward becoming a more experienced physician.

Being a patient turned out to be part of this journey, and having the tables turned on me was just one of the many unexpected lessons along the way. I realized that I would have to be alert to the rocks in the road and notice not just that they might hurt when stepped on, but that each would have a unique conformation, texture, and slope, and that each would leave a subtle yet distinctive imprint on me. If I wanted to learn from this voyage, I couldn't focus just on the ultimate goal of arrival; I'd have to pay careful attention the journey itself.

CHAPTER ONE

LIVING WILL

AFTER MY TEN YEARS OF MEDICAL SCHOOL and residency at New York City's Bellevue Hospital had finally ended, it took several weeks for my body to recover. And it took even longer for my mind. I couldn't quite believe that I would never again spend a night in a hospital. Never again find myself wandering deserted hallways at 3:00 in the morning. Never sweat over another IV in a veinless drug user. Never have to sleep in used sheets, shivering for lack of a blanket. And I would never again have to introduce myself as a doctor-in-training. I was finally a *real* doctor, whatever that meant.

After taking my internal medicine boards, my plan was to work for one month, then travel for as long as the money would last, then work again. A locum tenens agency set me up with assignments in various parts of the country, allowing me to fill in temporarily in clinics and hospitals.

My second temp agency assignment was in a small town on the Gulf Coast of Florida. I had only been working there for a few days when I received my first middle-of-the-night call from the hospital. In a daze I jotted down the information on the hotel stationery, then roused myself with cold water, hoping I would remember the directions to the hospital.

Wilbur Reston was already in the intensive care unit by the time I arrived at 2:30 A.M. The breathing tube in his throat and the heavy sedation precluded formal introductions. But there was a typewritten summary of his medical history that his wife had left with the nurses: a two-page, single-spaced odyssey that chronicled the rebellion and demise of each organ in this sixty-one-year-old white man. He had survived three heart attacks and seven strokes. One kidney had been removed. He suffered from diabetes, high blood pressure, and congestive heart failure. He had emphysema, glaucoma, severe migraines, and arthritis. His medical history included pancreatitis, diverticulitis, pyelonephritis, sinusitis, cholelithiasis, tinnitus, and ankylosing spondylitis. The typed paper also mentioned gastroesophageal reflux, vertigo, and depression. I quickly glanced over to the man hooked up to the ventilator to verify that he was indeed alive.

His wife had told the ER physicians that he'd stopped taking his water pills several days ago. Eventually he couldn't breathe. He possessed a living will stating that he did not want any life-sustaining procedures. In the ER, however, he had apparently agreed to be intubated. It had taken an enormous amount of sedation to get the breathing tube in, and as a result his blood pressure bottomed out. He was now unconscious in the ICU on multiple pressor medications to support his blood pressure and augment his weak heart. In the old Bellevue terminology, he was a train wreck.

Mr. Reston had been admitted to East General Hospital at 2:00 A.M. My colleagues in the small private practice where I was working had instructed me *never* to go to the hospital in the middle of the night. "Give your orders over the phone and see the patient in the morning," they advised. But I was still too new to this type of medicine to be that confident; I had to at least lay eyes on the patient before I could decide on any medical orders.

I couldn't take a history from Mr. Reston since he was, at present, unarousable due to all the sedation. My physical exam was brief. Mainly I plowed through the typed medical summary, converting it into a concise admission note. An hour later I handed my admitting orders to the nurse and then there was nothing for me to do. In this small community hospital, the nurses were used to and entirely comfortable with working without any doctors around. How unlike Bellevue, where interns and residents roamed the halls twenty-four hours a day, deeply and intricately involved in the minutiae of medical care. Here, the nurses took most of the doctors' orders over the phone and did everything themselves: drew blood, inserted IVs, did EKGs, obtained blood and urine cultures, sent patients for X-rays, followed up on test results, and performed myriad other tasks. The doctors, with their busy private practices, usually visited once a day, either very early in the morning or late, after their office hours. The emphasis was on remembering to sign the verbal orders within twenty-four hours. The head nurse was taken aback and almost alarmed when I showed up in the middle of the night for Mr. Reston's admission.

It was nearly four A.M. when I drove back to the hotel in my rental car. The main roads of the town were deserted. I rolled down the windows and was quickly enveloped in humid orange-scented fog. Stretches of flat, expressionless landscape were broken up by periodic strip malls. Low-slung houses of white stucco were interspersed with pickup trucks and palm trees. The smell of flower blossoms had not yet been fully eradicated by the burgeoning construction industry.

Southwest Florida was nothing like West Palm Beach, which I had assumed represented all of Florida. This area was rural, with acres of fields farmed by itinerant workers, mostly from Central America. I had just returned from Guatemala, so I was eager to practice my Spanish, but in the private practice where I worked, I rarely had the opportunity. Except for the time when I was called upon to explain to a Honduran fruit picker sitting in our waiting room that we couldn't treat his high blood pressure because he didn't have medical insurance. The hospital emergency room had called me when he'd shown up there needing prescriptions, and I said, Sure, send him over right now. When he arrived at the office, however, the practice manager curtly informed me that we could not treat such patients except in medical emergencies. Since I was the only one in the office who spoke passable Spanish, the duty of telling him fell to me.

My verb conjugations floundered and my pronouns violated their antecedents. My vocabulary in Spanish—and in English, for that matter—had never included such phrases as *We cannot take care of you. You must go to a different doctor.* I suddenly longed for Bellevue, for the chaos of its emergency room, with its bubbling tumult of languages, ethnicities, colors, and socioeconomic classes and its assumption that everybody received medical care regardless of ability to pay.

But aside from that one incident, the office was a pleasant place to work. Three doctors had started this practice several years ago and were now extremely successful. They had amassed an impressive roster of devoted patients, mainly older, but many middle-aged. They had equipped their office with a tiny pharmacy and a stress-test machine and had arranged for weekly visits from an ultrasound technician to do all their sonograms. They'd even opened a small gym next door in which they sponsored exercise classes for the elderly and rehab classes for their patients with emphysema. The doctors were in their forties, looking for ways to cut down on hours and enter semiretirement. They were more than happy to hand over a third of the office patients and 100 percent of the inpatient hospital duties. They gladly agreed to my request for paid preparation time, so that I could read patients' charts in advance of their appointments, all in a comfortable office with an experienced, full-time nurse to assist me. It was the lap of luxury. Within a week, they offered me a permanent, full-time position, with a salary that was four times what I'd earned as a resident for working half the hours, plus a share in the practice.

It all seemed too easy. The patients were pleasant and apparently particularly happy to have a woman doctor for the first time in that practice. And for the first time in *my* life, medicine was not a struggle: I could practice the best medicine I wanted without having to fight for anything. Coming from the trenches of Bellevue, where medicine often felt like warfare, the ease of practicing good medicine was almost disconcerting. I couldn't deny that the job offer was tempting.

But I could never move from Manhattan. Certainly not to live in such a tiny town.

The town was a speck on the map in southwest Florida that no one I knew had ever heard of. The pace was unhurried and the locals were unceasingly friendly and helpful, sometimes unsettlingly so to a native New Yorker. Overly polite strangers made me suspicious, though everyone assured me that this was the normal style in the South. There was no place to get sushi, but the two-room library across the street from my office did stock Spanish-lesson tapes, and I was able study a semester's worth of grammar on my way to work each day. Much to my dismay and disbelief, the library did not subscribe to the *New York Times*. A very weak consolation was the *Wall Street Journal*, which was only available, however, a day late.

The private practice was affiliated with East General, an eighty-eight-bed community hospital. I'd never seen a hospital that small. Eighty-eight beds was a single floor at Bellevue, and at Bellevue there were twenty-one floors. East General Hospital reminded me of my elementary school—spread out over two leggy wings, each only two stories high. The elevator seemed unnecessary. Some of the services that I was used to from Bellevue, like twenty-four-hour-a-day access to cardiac catheterization and hemodialysis, were not available, but there were advantages. With a maximum census of eighty-eight patients, there was never any waiting time for anything I ordered. Stress tests, sonograms, CT scans, pulmonary consults, social work requests—I had only to jot an order in the chart and it would be completed by the end of the day. The staff was small, but everyone seemed competent and extremely friendly. Within a week even the housekeepers were greeting me by name, and the phone operators recognized my voice when I called.

<hr />

The following morning Mr. Reston was awake but extremely uncomfortable. He had tried to pull out his breathing tube several times, so the nurses had tied down his arms. I apologized to him for the wrist restraints and explained that I would try to get the tube out as soon as possible. I was self-conscious about my words, because Wilbur Reston was sentient. He heard and understood everything I said, but the tube and the restraints prevented him from speaking or even gesturing in response. My reassurances stumbled off into the awkward air between us.

I spent the morning in the ICU weaning Mr. Reston off the ventilator and draining fluid from his lungs. When the nurses were rolling him over to change the sheets, he managed to dislodge his own breathing tube and set himself free. There is an entire scientific literature on the most appropriate time to extubate a patient, based on pulmonary-function tests, blood-gas values, and chest X-ray findings. But the Bellevue ICU aphorism was that a patient was ready to be extubated when he or she reached over and yanked out the damn tube. Mr. Reston proved this true; enough fluid had been removed from his lungs that he was able to breathe, if a bit huskily, without the tube. His condition was still tenuous, though, and he was too exhausted from his ordeal to talk much. I waited awhile for his wife to arrive, but she never showed up.

Thirty-six hours after his admission I was finally able to "meet" Mr. Reston. Wilbur Reston was a burly fellow who looked surprisingly robust for a patient sporting such a thick medical record. I would have expected a shriveled old man, but he had beefy arms and a hefty belly. There was a tattoo of an alligator on his left biceps. The ICU bed sagged slightly under his weight whenever he shifted or turned.

Mr. Reston's face was pulled low on his neck by meaty jowls, and dark bags weighed down his eyes. He'd lived his entire life in this small town on the west coast of Florida. He was a veteran of the Korean War, with a specialty in artillery. After the war he'd worked as a police officer and spent some time training guard dogs.

His voice was surprisingly soft and somewhat morose. In slow, deliberate utterances he described a lifetime of progressively declining health. His arthritic pains and severe headaches seemed to have taken a greater toll on his life than his many strokes and heart attacks. He was confined to his house, unable even to walk down the driveway to retrieve his mail.

Did he have any hobbies? He heaved a melancholic sigh. "I fancied myself a carpenter. I built miniature furniture for dollhouses. Always used the best wood."

I imagined this bearlike man hunched over delicate divans and bedroom sets. "Can't do it anymore. My hands." He threw up his gnarled arthritic paws for inspection. "I also collect Civil War memorabilia. Once found a belt buckle from the Second Battle of Bull Run," he said, with a small puff of pride. "They had it in the museum for a while." But the recollection of his former glory was brief. "My wife thinks it's a stupid hobby."

What about depression? "I've never *not* been depressed." He sighed ruefully. "Ever since college, I suppose." His records showed that he'd been treated at the VA psychiatric clinic with both psychotherapy and antidepressant medications for more than twenty years. His only daughter had died of a brain tumor the year before. His mother and sister had both died in the past five years. So had his dog.

Had he ever attempted suicide? "I'm handy with guns, you know. I have at least five in the house," he said dryly. "Different models. Always keep a loaded one at my bedside." Did he ever use it? "Well, I stuck the barrel in my mouth once. Didn't pull the trigger, though. Too messy. Just stopped taking my pills."

I had an image of Mr. Reston sitting on the side of his bed, shoulders sagging, cradling the gun in his hand. Perhaps he'd raised the gun to his head several times, each time not able to summon it close enough. But then he'd take a quick dry swallow, and, squinting his eyes shut, will his hand aloft with sheer inner power. Then he would slide the gun into his mouth. The cool metal would press easily past his chapped lips and come to rest within the softness of his cheek and tongue. I imagined that he might be startled at how comforting the gun felt in his mouth. But then that very comfort would make him shudder, and he'd rip the gun out, stuff it back into the nightstand drawer, and slam the drawer shut.

Then he'd be left staring at the pill bottles lined up like mercenaries on that nightstand, their chambers loaded with bullet-size promises of good health. He'd finger them, recalling what ill each was meant to treat. And treat they did. And then what?

I envisioned him opening that drawer again, and with a harsh flick of his clublike arm, sweeping the bottles in, their hard plastic armor clattering against the gun as they came to rest at the bottom. He'd sink his head into his hands, forgetting to shut the nightstand drawer.

What about his wife? "She's busy with that volunteer work. She don't have time for me and all my pills," he said sadly.

An uneasy silence settled in. I could see moisture accumulating on the edges of his soulful eyes. "We haven't shared a bed in fifteen years," he whispered.

His voice was plaintive but resigned. "Why should I live this life? I can't walk, my wife don't speak to me, I can't do nothing. What's the point?" He fixed his mournful gaze upon me. "*You* tell *me*."

It was both a plea and a demand. His simple statement evaporated the space between us, and I suddenly felt naked. Without my clinical armor to shield me, I was just one human facing another, squinting before the raw question. What *was* the point? What were the reasons for him to go on living?

I struggled to come up with one. Mr. Reston's body had withered sufficiently to keep him in perpetual pain but not enough to let him die. He had no friends; his wife was estranged. His daughter, mother, and sister had died, abandoning him. He was too weak to walk out of his house. He could no longer do any of the things that brought him pleasure. Why should he want to live? I could see why he had stopped taking his pills.

I didn't have an answer for him, but the law dictated what I had to do: actively suicidal patients must be prevented from harming themselves. Like all good emergencies, this one occurred late on a Friday afternoon. Unlike Bellevue, there was no residency program in psychiatry to supply round-the-clock consultations. There were several psychiatrists in the community, but they were busy with their private practices during the day and rarely made after-hours calls.

But the staff of this tiny hospital was resourceful and helpful. They got me in touch with the local mental-health agency, which was able to dispatch a psychiatric nurse practitioner. She agreed with my concerns and helped the nursing staff arrange a one-to-one suicide watch over Mr. Reston. I could transfer Mr. Reston to a psychiatric hospital once his medical condition stabilized if I felt he was still in danger of hurting himself. The nurse practitioner explained the procedures to invoke the Baker Act, the state legislation that allowed involuntary psychiatric commitment in such circumstances.

Over that weekend Mr. Reston's medical condition slowly improved, but his mood did not. Why should it? I thought. What did he have to look forward to? As much as I tried, I could not bring myself to utter flimsy platitudes about the value of life and how things would be better tomorrow. They weren't going to get better—he knew it and I knew it. Although he was clearly depressed, Mr. Reston was perfectly lucid. Despite his many strokes, his mind seemed to be working just fine. He could do all the tasks in the mental status exam: spell *world* backward, count down from 100 by sevens, name the president, interpret the saying "A rolling stone gathers no moss."

Although Mr. Reston seemed to have a reasonably realistic grasp on his situation, I wasn't so sure if I had a grasp on mine. Doctors aren't supposed to agree with their patients when they say they want to kill themselves, but I found myself overwhelmed by the utterly dismal facts of Mr. Reston's life. I could never live his life. If every pleasure disappeared and every person I loved was gone, I didn't think I could go on living. What did Mr. Reston have left to live for? Even his dog had died.

I tried to imagine pacing the blank landscape of an empty life, wandering among hollow structures from which all my loved ones had melted away. How could I survive if every source of pleasure was denied by the intransigence of my body and the unforgivingness of my environment? How could I live if the flavors, colors, and textures that made life palatable were flattened into a monochrome gray? If I were Mr. Reston, I might have pulled that trigger.

To complicate matters, Mr. Reston was in a rather unique medical situation. Although he had multitudes of medical problems, he was not terminally ill. He was sick enough to be miserable, but not sick enough to die. He was still able to eat, care for himself, and communicate with others. There were plenty of services and options for people on the verge of death, but Mr. Reston was not sick enough to qualify. His body, honed from years in the military and police force, was holding on too tenaciously. It left him in the miserable muck, stranded too far from the shores of either health or death.

Mr. Reston had severe physical pain, apparently unresponsive to various treatments, but more important, he was being eaten away by psychic pain. He had been ravaged by his own life and was left with only a shell of himself. Insidious emotional torment had battered his heart as much as the atherosclerotic plaques had.

The medicolegal issues were clear: a suicidal patient is prevented, even against his will, from committing suicide, period. But the shades of gray needled me: my patient didn't want his life, and I wasn't sure if it was ethical to force him to continue living it.

These issues plagued me for the remainder of the week. Ashamed to reveal my heresies to anyone, I secretly toyed with my doubts, poking at them as one does a loose tooth, perversely finding pleasure in its pain. What if I let him go home to his household of loaded guns? What if I discharged him, knowing full well that he'd stop taking his life-saving medicines? What if I turned my head and let him kill himself as he so desperately wanted to do? There are those who say that all suicidal thoughts are products of depression, but Mr. Reston had been assiduously treated with medications and psychotherapy for decades. Perhaps he was being entirely rational. Who was I to stand in his way?

Then the toothache would burrow down to the raw nerve: What kind of evil doctor was I even to *consider* not protecting my patient from his violent tendencies? How could I be so negligent?

As I drove back and forth to work each day, this dilemma nagged at me. Lulled by the bland landscape, my mind would wander from the Spanish vocabulary emanating from the car's tape deck to Mr. Reston languishing in his bare hospital room. Could there ever be any happiness for him? What if I found him a new hobby, one that he could manage with his disabilities? Stamp collecting—that wouldn't require much mobility. But probably his fingers couldn't manipulate the fragile paper stamps. Maybe he could take up painting. Large easy brushes with big tubs of paint—he could manage that. Maybe he'd discover bold strokes of color, thick swaths of pigment layering on taut canvas. Perhaps there was an artist waiting inside his battle-weary body.

Traffic was stopped as a cumbersome tractor-trailer backed out of a dirt construction site, attempting to turn itself around. A grove of orange trees had just been plowed, probably to make way for a new strip mall. The trailer was open on top, and I could see the stacks of shimmering steel girders. The driver backed up a few feet, and then the trailer swung in the opposite direction, blocking his turn. The workers on the road waved their hands, shouting contradictory instructions: "Pull back a bit." "Swing to the right." "Turn your wheels on a sharp left." The driver edged forward and back, craning his neck out the window then up toward his rearview mirror as he tried to extricate himself from the tight spot. The steel girders flashed in the sunlight each time he changed angles. The smell of fresh damp earth blended with the intoxicating sweetness of the orange blossoms, something I'd never smelled in New York City.

The metallic clanking and the competing shouts, along with the glare of the sunlight and the overpowering fragrance, made me feel queasy and somewhat faint. I leaned my head against the steering wheel, when suddenly I saw the hole in Mr. Reston's armor: he had let himself be intubated. This man who possessed a living will explicitly refusing all life-sustaining procedures had *voluntarily* allowed a breathing tube to force air into his drowning lungs. He had reached for a life preserver.

I picked my head up, feeling the murkiness begin to clear. Despite all of Wilbur Reston's misgivings and doubts, a desire to live had percolated through.

As I leaned back in my seat, I wondered how that had come to pass. Was it simply the life-grabbing instinct that springs forward in such moments of near-doom? Or was it truly evidence of Mr. Reston's ambivalence, of a desire to be saved and cared for?

Clearly, I had no way to know—I doubted if he himself even knew—but it seemed to me that Mr. Reston had given himself permission for a second chance. Now that he had done so, I had the opportunity, perhaps even the obligation, to allow that chance to flourish. If this second chance wasn't nourished, there probably wouldn't be a third.

The tractor-trailer veered to the left and finally pulled itself out of its trap. The traffic snarl cleared and I jammed on the accelerator, flying down the road with the breath of orange blossoms sweeping against my face.

—————

When his medical condition stabilized, Mr. Reston was involuntarily committed to a VA psychiatric facility. He didn't protest when I informed him. He just nodded his head, his baggy jowls bobbing. During his entire stay, I'd never once met his wife; her occasional visits never seemed to coincide with mine.

The VA doctors assumed care of Mr. Reston, and I had no more contact. The private practice was busy and I saw many patients each day. My mind was filled with Shana Elron's brittle diabetes and Henry Shaw's uncontrolled hypertension. And there was the lady with pneumonia whom I was trying to keep out of the hospital and the gentleman with emphysema who was finally willing to try giving up cigarettes. There was the couple who lived in

Pennsylvania during the summer but spent winters down south, and I was helping them coordinate his prostate cancer treatment between the two locations. I had recommitted myself to Spanish and spent my evenings conjugating verbs. I planned to leave for Mexico as soon as this stint in Florida was over, and I wanted to have the conditional tense under my belt. I had to decide if I wanted to start my trip in Guadalajara and end in Chiapas or vice versa. Or maybe just fly straight to Oaxaca and enroll in the Spanish school there. And then there was that shell-beach peninsula set against a tangle of mangroves twenty minutes from my hotel that beckoned me every night after work. I soon forgot about Mr. Reston.

Several weeks later, as my assignment in Florida was drawing to a close, some paperwork concerning Mr. Reston's original hospital admission turned up in my office, requiring a signature. Wilbur Reston's morose face flickered in my mind and I thought about his miniature doll furniture. I wished I were still his doctor.

Besides giving himself a second chance, Mr. Reston had granted me the opportunity to tease out some of the more subtle aspects of medicine. He forced me to see beyond his imposing resume of disease, beyond his exhaustively documented medical pathologies, to his simple, hurting human self. The patient is not simply the sum of his illnesses, Wilbur Reston taught me. It is far more—blessedly far more—intricate than that.

After negotiating a labyrinth of phone calls through the VA bureaucracy I finally tracked down his psychiatrist. Mr. Reston had been discharged just a few days ago. The psychiatrist described the long weeks and the laborious effort it had required to get Mr. Reston to take responsibility for simple things like brushing his teeth. By the end, though, he was showing up at the group meetings, even if he rarely spoke. Once in a while he even went to arts and crafts. Mr. Reston did not become an effusive, energetic person, but according to the psychiatrist he no longer actively expressed the wish to die. That was considered a major success. And once he was no longer suicidal, there was no justification for keeping him involuntarily hospitalized. He could go home to his wife and continue with his regular outpatient therapy.

The psychiatrist commiserated with me over the many painful but immutable realities of Mr. Reston's life. A social worker was trying to help Mr. Reston get a new dog—that was about the only thing they could remedy.

I flew to Mexico the following week. In the end I decided to fly directly to Oaxaca for a month of Spanish lessons. Afterward I'd trek to Chiapas to see the Mayan ruins. I plunged into my classes, determined not to speak a word of English for six weeks if that was possible. I rented a room from a family that spoke no English; I purchased Spanish editions of *Jonathan Livingston Seagull* and *The Little Prince* as my reading material; I tried to minimize my social contacts with the other foreigners in my classes and, instead, hang out at local cafés.

But I still thought about Wilbur Reston and wondered how he was doing. Those thoughts could only be in English. I imagined that he was sitting alone in his house, his wife at yet another volunteer function, his bones still aching, his weak heart preventing him from even getting the mail. But maybe there was now a puppy yapping at his feet, freely dispensing and demanding love. When the headaches and joint pains became overwhelming, maybe Mr. Reston would again consider ending his life. But then he might stop and think: Who would feed the puppy?

CHAPTER TWO

COMMON GROUND

"WE *ARE* A CATHOLIC MEDICAL CENTER, Dr. Ofri." The medical director leaned back in his chair across from my desk. "Do you have any issues with that?"

His gray hair was severely parted on the right and I could trace the individual strands that were tethered down on the side by hair grease. A stethoscope peeked out of the pocket of his tailored blue suit. He had just finished his long introductory speech, enumerating the vast array of services and the selling points of his medical group. He was clearly trying to impress me with his institution. After all, the reason I was doing a temp assignment here was that they were short-handed and looking to hire.

I was caught off balance by the question. What could he be driving at? Was my Jewish background an issue here? Was my last name too "ethnic"? I paused and then slowly asked, "*Should* I have issues?"

"Well," he replied in his careful New England lilt, "we do not promote birth control. If a patient requests it, we will provide it. But we do not offer it, promote it, or condone it."

Before my superego could grab control, my New York sassiness spilled out. "So I don't suppose you perform abortions, do you." I could not believe I had just said that.

The older physician did not appear fazed. "No, we do not terminate pregnancies. Nor do we allow referrals to physicians who do. If a patient requests that service, we have them call their own insurance company. Their insurance companies make the referral."

He stood up and put out his hand. "We are glad to have you aboard, Dr. Ofri. We hope you enjoy your six weeks with us. And" —he paused with a smile— "we hope you will consider staying longer."

I had never spent much time in New England before. The town looked just as I had imagined it would. Regal Victorian mansions with wraparound wooden porches lined the main street. Well-tended rosebushes graced the picket fences. Manicured shrubbery lined the driveways. A river meandered through the town and I often saw kayakers as I drove over the small bridges each morning in my beige rental car.

There was a small-town civility that was quite different than my native New York and was certainly a world apart from the boisterous, colorful chaos of Mexico. For the past month I'd immersed myself in Spanish conjugations, poblano chilies, Neruda poems, and guava milkshakes in the southern city of Oaxaca. Spanish classes were in the mornings, and the afternoons were for exploring. The streets of Oaxaca were paved with pale yellow limestone that reminded me of Jerusalem. It was a cosmopolitan city of museums and universities, but it was also filled with ethnic diversity from the surrounding villages. On weekends I boarded the second-class buses with the local villagers and their children and their chickens and traveled to the different villages. The fringed curtains in the bus windows and the dangling icons of the Virgin of Guadalupe on the rearview mirrors fluttered in the wind as we jostled along the dirt roads. Each village specialized in a particular craft. There was the village of the green pottery, which was distinct from the village of the black pottery. There was the village of the painted wooden animals and the village of the woven rugs. I wandered from house to house, perusing the handicrafts displayed on the patios, trying out my newly acquired verbs. Most people were friendly and indulged my mangling of their language.

Oaxaca was also known for its diverse cuisine. The specialties were spicy chocolate mole and *chapulines* (fried grasshoppers) served with chili and lime. I sampled the former, which I found too rich and too sweet, but never quite got to the latter. My personal culinary epiphany came when I discovered the sublime mango-con-chili-flavored ice pop. The sweet frozen treat with a zap of chili was the perfect antidote to the hot, dusty days. My fingers were stained rusty orange for the duration of my trip. To this day I can't fathom why my fellow Americans have never caught on to the joy of chili on sweets.

When my money supply ran low, I called my locum tenens agency. Luckily, they accepted collect calls from Latin America, and they had arranged this job assignment for me in New England.

I was assigned to a small private practice that was short-handed after two doctors had moved away. The staff members welcomed me warmly. They gave me a large office with three exam rooms in a separate wing of the suite. Karen, an exceptionally talented nurse, was assigned to work exclusively with me. The receptionists consulted with me each day to ensure that my schedule had no conflicts. The office manager checked in periodically to make sure that all my needs were met. Like my experience in Florida, practicing medicine had never been so easy.

I noticed that the medicine cabinet was stocked with free samples of birth control pills along with the antihypertensives and cholesterol-lowering medications. Apparently, the contraception rule wasn't taken too seriously.

The patients who came to this practice were friendly and seemed happy to have a new doctor available. Most were of French-Canadian descent. Their families had emigrated more than two generations ago, so their French-spelled last names were pronounced with a decidedly American twang. St. Denis and du Maurier, as I recalled from my college days in Montreal, were supposed to lilt off the tongue, only barely touching down at the ends: "san de-Nee" and "du mawr-Yay." Here in New England they were plodded out with equal and literal emphasis on every syllable: "Saint Den-nis" and "Doo-maw-ree-yare."

Karen was a dream to work with. At the beginning of each appointment she would obtain a brief history from the patient, check the vital signs, and jot down the medications. When I entered the room afterward, I would find all the supplies that I might need for that particular patient, based on Karen's initial interview, neatly laid out. I learned that the walls of the examining rooms were fairly thin, because when I was finished with the patient, Karen would be waiting outside with whatever vaccines or medications had been discussed. And I loved that she kept a picture of her golden retriever, Sam, on her desk.

Karen and I occupied a private wing of the office. Nobody ever bothered us in our little corner. Between patients we would share stories of her life in New England and my experiences in Mexico. She told me where the least stuffy restaurants could be found and which parks had free Shakespeare plays. I told her about sharing a seat with three turkeys on a six-hour bus ride over the Oaxacan mountains to the seaside town of Puerto Escondido. I related some of my tales from Bellevue, the colorfully psychotic patients in the ER, and medical dramas in the ICU. She helped me plan for my upcoming trip to Peru. We leafed through the travel book, debating between Cusco and Arequipa for my next Spanish class. We worked so smoothly together that the days sped effortlessly along.

Three weeks into my assignment I met Diana Rakower, a young computer programmer at a local financial firm. She was wearing a gray suit with a purple silk blouse. A single strand of pearls dipped around her neck. Her carefully applied makeup had started to smudge from the tears slipping down her cheeks. "I think I'm pregnant," she spilled out almost before I could introduce myself. "I did one of those home pregnancy tests and it was positive. All I need from you is the blood test to confirm."

I put down my stethoscope and pulled up a chair.

"It's a complicated situation," she wept. "I am ending a relationship with my boyfriend, but it wasn't him. I have an old friend, it's never been more than that, but I think he and I might be developing a romantic relationship. We slept together just once, three weeks ago. I really think we could have a serious relationship, but it is not ready for this. I can't believe this is happening."

"If you do turn out to be pregnant," I asked, "what do you think you would do?"

"I need to end it. I can't have a kid now; I'm single, I don't have a stable relationship yet. I'm not ready for it now."

"Are you sure that's what you want to do? Have you considered other options, like adoption? "

"Absolutely," she said. "I have made my decision. I just need to know where to go."

I suddenly thought of the medical director with his slicked-down gray hair. According to the rules, I was supposed to tell Diana to call her insurance company.

Her insurance company? I had visions of a bored bureaucrat slurping on his coffee while dispensing advice on a delicate matter to my distraught patient. How could I send Diana into a situation like that? I excused myself and went to consult Karen.

Karen did not know which local doctors performed abortions. The Catholic hospital that the practice was affiliated with certainly did not. "I stay out of that mess," she said. She sympathized with my predicament but warned me not to let the office manager know what I was doing. "Someone else gave out a phone number once," she said, "just a phone number. It wasn't even documented in the chart, but somehow it got out and they got into trouble."

I stared out the window and could see my rental car parked in front of a clapboard house across the street. The house was painted bright yellow with pale blue trim. A wooden porch surrounded three sides of the house. An American flag dangled from a second-story window. This Catholic medical institution might choose not to perform abortions, but what about *my* ethical duty to provide the care my patient needed? Sending a distressed patient to a toll-free phone number seemed like a dereliction of duty.

It seemed clear to me that my duty was first to my patient and only second to some faceless institution. Unfortunately, as a stranger to this small town, I did not know the local resources. I didn't know the names of nearby physicians to refer her to, even if I wanted to break the rules. I looked back at the yellow and blue house across the road. It seemed hostile and antagonistic. The small-town civility made me feel claustrophobic.

Grinding my teeth, I reentered the exam room. "As you may know, this medical practice is Catholic," I told Diana, "so we cannot provide referrals for abortion. The truth is, I wouldn't know where to send you even if I could. The rule is that you are supposed to call your insurance company and get the referral yourself. I would do it for you, but I don't think the insurance company would allow me to. However, if you get a list of possible referrals, I will call around to find out which is the best."

Diana nodded and then asked if she could be alone. I left her with a box of tissues and told her she could stay as long as she liked.

I phoned Diana the next day to let her know that the repeat pregnancy test was positive. When I called, I got her voice mail at work. She had told me that it was a private line, but suddenly I felt paranoid. I did not indicate that I was a physician and I left a cryptic message about results being "confirmatory of our original data."

Diana returned my call a few hours later. Her insurance company had given her two phone numbers, without names, in the next state over. Her health plan had no gynecologists in this state who performed abortions.

Nobody in the state? My patient couldn't get the care that she needed in her home state? I was horrified. How could I send her off into the unknown like that? How could I abandon her to a couple of random, blank telephone numbers in another state? I felt like we were back in the 1950s, sneaking around with code words, no names mentioned, having to go out of state for an abortion.

I plowed through my roster of patients for the day, but I couldn't focus on the coughs, rashes, and shoulder pains. All I could think about was Diana. I imagined her driving over the state line, tears pressing at her lid margins. The lonesomeness in the car, the bitter highway, the directions scribbled on the back of a used envelope. I imagined her squinting at the scrawled directions, the car slipping ever so slightly in the lane as her mind diffused focus from the highway median to those directions specifying the second left after the traffic light to the enormity of what lay ahead. Between patients I paced around my office, too irritated to sit still. What kind of place was this where some administrative rule could interfere with patient care? Wasn't patient care more important than a bunch of rules?

When was the last time any of those bureaucrats actually *saw* a patient? When was the last time they'd sat face-to-face with a woman, watching the tension lines around her mouth quiver, smelling the moist desperation, accepting the burden and the honor of tender secrets? I fumed all afternoon, cursing the insurance companies and the politicians whose ideologies and business concerns were elbowing into my office, into the sacred space that my patient and I shared.

Then Karen told me that the wife of one of the doctors used to work at a teen clinic. Grateful for this information, I called immediately. She knew of those two out-of-state facilities and told me they had reputations for treating patients like cattle. There was, however, a private women's clinic two hours north that was both professional and reliable. But most insurance companies would not cover the cost of the procedure.

I called Diana at home that evening. She had already made an appointment at one of the out-of-state clinics and was very appreciative of my insider information. I gave her the number of the private women's clinic.

"Have you told him?" I asked.

"No. No, I can't tell him. Not yet, at least. Maybe afterward."

"Is there anyone that you'd feel comfortable talking to—a

friend, a family member? Is there someone who could come with you?"

"No, not really," she replied. "I mean, I have good friends, but I couldn't tell them about this. They wouldn't understand."

I winced at the thought of her going alone. There was a sense of something shameful, something to hide. "Bring your own bathrobe," I added before we hung up. "It's more comfortable than a hospital gown."

I called her again the following day, just to make sure she was okay. We chatted a bit and it turned out that she had grown up in New York.

"Really?" I asked, excited to uncover a fellow New York native here in the wilds of New England. "Where were you born?"

"Queens," she said, "but then we moved out to Long Island, which is where I really grew up."

"My family did something similar. I was born in Manhattan but then we moved out of the city. I hated the suburbs, though. I think I never forgave my parents for leaving the city."

"Me too," Diana said. "I spent all of my high school years hanging out in Greenwich Village, trying to make up for my parents' foolish flight to the 'burbs."

"So did I," I said excitedly. "We used to tramp up and down Bleeker Street buying earrings and incense from street vendors, then go hear music at Kenny's Castaways."

"I know Kenny's Castaways," she said. "The club that never checked ID."

"That's the one. And you went to Le Figaro Café, didn't you?"

"Absolutely—southeast corner of Bleeker and MacDougal. That's where I had my first cappuccino. I couldn't bear to drink my parents' instant coffee after that."

I left work that evening and drove home to my hotel. The very act of driving, of commuting by car—something I was forced to do during these locum tenens assignments in small towns—made me feel odd. In Montreal there was the Metro. In New York I'd been a regular denizen of the subway, a regular, that is, until I discovered the superior efficiency and enjoyment of a bicycle.

My bicycle could take me anywhere in New York City. With a Kryptonite lock and a cardboard box strapped on the back, I could cycle through the cultures and generations of the world. Middle Eastern markets, Ethiopian restaurants, Jamaican neighborhoods were all accessible. I biked to a wetlands preserve in Queens, an old waterfront farmhouse in Staten Island, the Hasidic neighborhoods of Brooklyn, a seventeenth-century Sephardic cemetery in Manhattan. All I needed was a picnic lunch in the cardboard box on the back of my bike and at least one section of the *New York Times*, and I could spend the day anywhere. Only major snowstorms and pouring rain drove me to unearth my subway tokens and go underground.

And now I sat in my car, cut off from humanity, isolated in a metal box that rumbled with diesel heat under my feet as the traffic light languished on red. Sure, the old houses were beautiful to look at and the landscaping impressive, but there were no people on the street, no people walking around. Only cars.

Stuck in my car, my mind stayed with Diana, and I was reminded of sitting in a similar traffic jam thinking about Wilbur Reston. It seemed that three-ton hulks of steel were somehow conducive to reflection. Diana was also cut off. There was no one, apparently, in whom she could confide, no one she could bring with her. I realized that I was probably the only person in this world she had spoken to about this. In the tiny, enclosed space of my car, with that bland smell of whatever they use to make seat stuffing, the heaviness of that burden weighed on the cramped muscles of my shoulders. There were hundreds of people tucked into similar steel automobiles who were riding along the same street as I was, hundreds of cars shuttling human beings within their tiny isolated orbits, but only one that contained Diana Rakower's confidence.

As a woman, I felt an almost sisterly duty to be there for her during this uniquely female quandary. As her doctor, I felt that I had the responsibility to make sure she got the medical care she needed and felt guilty that I couldn't help her more directly. And as a human being, I felt the moral obligation to treat that confidence with the utmost respect. I couldn't abandon her during this difficult and lonely period.

When I arrived back at my hotel, I called her again, just to see how she was doing. Two days later I called Diana again. I somehow found a pretext to call her almost every day until her abortion date the following week.

I felt a bit more like a therapist than a physician and I understood why therapists are to keep their personal lives out of the therapy. Therapy is about the patient, not about the therapist.

I ached to share my own experience, but professionalism, and I suppose some lingering shame, prevented me. I'd been only seventeen at the time and just returning home from my first year in college. I had passed my calculus final exam and was fairly confident about physics. I had turned in my last organic chemistry lab report. I was about to go off to be a counselor at summer camp when I discovered that I was pregnant.

I'd had a steady boyfriend the entire year. Before we'd gotten involved, I had gone to Planned Parenthood because I didn't want to be irresponsible. I remembered the long talk with the counselor in the windowless room with the cheery posters. We'd decided together on the diaphragm for birth control. The package insert listed a 95 percent effectiveness rate.

No one ever spoke about the other 5 percent.

I lived in New York, the most liberal city in the most liberal state. My friends and parents were all liberal, pro-choice people. But I was too scared to tell anyone. It just didn't seem possible that it was happening and it didn't seem possible to tell anyone.

After the pregnancy test, I sat in a park and cried alone. It was a park where my family used to have picnics when I was little. My parents would buy a roasted chicken from the nearby kosher deli.

We'd bring paper plates and the vegetable salad. And of course, our beloved mutt, Kushi. This was her chance to run off the leash. Sitting in that park now I longed for the smell of her soft black fur. I craved her warm, all-accepting dogness to snuggle up to.

I arranged an appointment at a local women's clinic. That night I made a long-distance call to my boyfriend. The geographical and personal gaps were apparently too vast to bridge—he couldn't quite accept what I was telling him over the phone. And he didn't offer to help me pay for it.

The next day I lied to my parents about having a party to go to so I could borrow the car. The clinic said to bring a comfortable bathrobe. I snuck my mother's out of her closet.

The drive was eerily dissociated. The yellow lines in the road didn't seem parallel to the outer curbs. They listed and buckled, slighting the rules of Cartesian geometry. They drifted to other planes, to the odd dimensions of irrational numbers. Then they'd swing back with a jolt, clobbering into my focus. As the car shuffled closer and closer to the clinic, I felt my body shrinking. It dwindled within itself until there was nothing left but a little girl who desperately wanted her dog.

I lugged myself, or what little was left of myself, up the steps. I registered and followed the nurse into the back. She instructed me to change into my bathrobe and wait in the main room until I was called. The room was filled with eight women in different-colored bathrobes. We could have been at a slumber party, except that no one was smiling. Some magazines were scattered on the table, but the articles were about beef casseroles and electricity-saving tips. I tugged my mother's flannel robe tighter around me and concentrated on the orange industrial carpeting. It really was orange, although if you looked carefully, there were lonely bits of red and yellow scattered within.

They gave me a choice of general or local anesthesia. The budding scientist wanted local anesthesia, wanted to know everything that was going on, wanted to control the whole biology experiment. But the little girl who yearned for her dog immediately chose general anesthesia. I didn't want to know. I didn't want to remember.

I awoke crying in another room. It was overly bright and the sheets were stiff. My stomach pulsed with an alien ache. The nurse said to stop acting like a baby, it didn't really hurt that much. I checked out and went back to the same park to cry some more.

A week later, a letter arrived from my boyfriend. He told me that he felt terribly guilty. As "penance" for himself, he said he could never be with me again.

That summer was long and lonely.

In the years that have gone by I have told almost no one. Part of me feels that I should be contributing to the destigmatization of abortion by being open about my own experience. Yet another part of me feels that it is something personal. Worse yet, something to hide. I feel guilty and hypocritical.

Sometimes I think about the child that might have been. At seventeen, I had precious few resources to raise a child. I would never have finished college, much less gone to medical school. I might have faced a lifetime of minimum-wage jobs and food stamps. What would my child's life have been like?

I called Diana after her abortion. She told me that the staff members at the clinic were extremely kind and supportive, and that it didn't hurt too much. I breathed a sigh of relief. We spoke a few more times after that. Each time I felt the urge to share my story, but I couldn't.

I am not a particularly politically active person. So much of what transpires in the government seems to have no bearing on my life; I just want to take care of my patients and my family. The decision about abortion is a difficult one, not one that I would wish anyone to face. A different time or a different place and the outcome could have been vastly different. I often think of the sad eyes and weary wrinkles of Dr. Weisner, the elderly gynecology professor who'd told us medical students of having to lug young, bleeding women up the stone staircases of Bellevue during his internship. "You kids don't remember," he said in a soft, reflective voice. "You kids just don't know what it was like."

When I see teenage mothers in my clinic with minimal education, no job skills, barely mature enough to take care of themselves, let alone the two or three babies on their laps, I am viscerally aware that my life was at the mercy of laws that permitted access to safe abortion.

Doctors often unconsciously separate themselves from patients—*they* are the sick ones and *we*, in our white coats, are different from them. It is humbling, and also relieving, to know that we are all made of the same stuff.

CHAPTER THREE

ACNE

A YOUNG NAVAJO WOMAN files silently into my office, making no eye contact. As she slips into the chair errant strands of black hair spill across her face. Through the breaches I catch glimpses of her rich dark skin riddled with the pockmarks of severe acne. Violently swollen pustules and angry red craters contort the architecture of her face. Her shoulders slope into her slight body, as if afraid to claim too much territory on their own. She contemplates the linoleum wordlessly. I am almost afraid to interrupt.

I am not her regular physician. At this clinic she has no regular physician because of high turnover and a chronic shortage of doctors. I myself am just a temp, a hired hand deposited briefly in this small New Mexican town.

I ask my patient what brings her here. She quietly lays out her litany of symptoms: fatigue, headaches, stomach pains, and her worsening skin condition. I leaf through her clinic chart as she speaks and I can see that over the years acne has been her major problem. It is repeatedly noted that she cannot afford to see a dermatologist for specialty treatment.

Almost perfunctorily I ask my usual question about the presence of stress in her life. Almost as perfunctorily she replies that her husband hanged himself two months ago. One month prior he had made a first suicide attempt. Their twelve-year-old son discovered him hanging and untied the rope. The father was furious and beat the boy. Four weeks later, the father found the rope his son had dutifully hidden and hanged himself again, this time successfully.

My patient remains impassive as she relates this tale to me. This is where he hit me the first time, she says, raising her sleeve above her elbow. The beer bottle was already broken when he hit me so it left a scar.

I lean over to look where she is pointing—the purple scar is jagged and raised. It has pulled the skin around it into an ugly pucker. The harshly engraved lines remind me of the craggy desert landscape that I see everyday as I drive to work in this tiny, dusty town. I can feel a dry heat emanating from where she points.

It doesn't show on the stomach, she says in her unembellished monotone, but I still get pains here. She hoists her cotton shirt up and I see golden skin with faint stretch marks. When I was pregnant I tried not to let him kick me there, but it was hard sometimes.

I don't see scars but my ears pound with screams.

I had my tubes tied, she says, but he was mad. He wanted more kids. I thought two was enough, but he wanted more. A real Navajo tribe, was what he said. She intertwines one finger in an ebony lock of hair. Her voice continues—flatly, plainly. He got drunk a lot more then. He wanted me to do another operation. To untie them. It's not that I don't like kids—I love my boys—but I wasn't sure if we should have any more. Kids are expensive. She rotates her finger and the hair twists with it, glistening under the pale office lights. I am beginning to perspire in this overly air-conditioned room.

Almost a year we argued about it, she says. We had some bad fights. But I finally decided to do it, untie them. I do like kids. I made an appointment at the hospital for the surgery, but he was mad because it wasn't soon enough. Then he killed himself.

I try to respond matter-of-factly, wanting to put her at ease, but I am assaulted by the vision of a man hanging and a young child stumbling into the room. Was the body writhing in agony? Was the face exploding with hypoxic torment? What did it look like from twelve-year-old eyes? What could it feel like to unhitch a rope from a dying man's neck?

What about my acne, she asks. Can't anything be done?

For a moment I can only blink dumbly at her, fixated on the web that extends far beyond this office and the capabilities of the medical profession. I hunger for powers to untangle the knots, but medical school has not made me a healer of all pains. The illusion of omniscience blithely promised by my residency training is easily deflated by the unadorned actualities of life. Her acne is all I *can* attack, though I see that physicians here before me have waged this war without success.

Surveying her medical history penned by so many different hands, I observe that she has tried most of the basic acne medications. There is one, however, that she has not taken. It is rarely prescribed to women of childbearing age because of its toxic effects on fetuses. Each individual capsule brandishes the image of a pregnant woman with an ominous X slashed through the swollen belly. But my patient's plans to reverse her tubal ligation were aborted by circumstance.

This medication is not available in our meager clinic pharmacy, and my patient does not have the means to obtain it on the outside. I have been told that drug companies will occasionally provide medications without charge. The bureaucracy can be arduous and there is no guarantee of success, but I think we should try. My patient agrees.

I observe in her chart that she has not had a recent Pap smear. I offer her the option of seeing the gynecologist but she prefers that I perform it, at our next visit. I am honored.

I watch her pad silently down the hall. Weakly, I retreat to my office. The stout medical textbooks and cabinets overflowing with equipment are stifling, mocking. Where did I get the absurd notion that I might be a healer?

When my month is up, I will move on. Just one in a stream of doctors, I, too, will abandon this young woman, bequeathing her only a bottle of pills. I scribble a note to call the drug company and then tape it to my bag. I cannot afford to forget.

CHAPTER FOUR

A Day in the Clinic

In some ways Bellevue is exactly as I left it. The same ivy-covered, nineteenth-century brick Old Bellevue building leads into the plain concrete New Bellevue. But the entranceway to the building has been given one facelift and is now in the process of a second. The grimy single-door entrance that crammed generations of Bellevue patients and employees into a bottleneck, forcing them through a narrow path under the dingy concrete overhang of the parking garage, has been boarded up. In its place was built a wide red-brick boulevard, covered by an arched glass roof through which the trees and sun are visible.

On First Avenue, at the beginning of the pathway to this new entrance, a massive concrete portal was erected, a replica of the original gate from 1811. It depicted a pilgrim and a Native American, presumably the local New Yorkers when Bellevue Hospital was first established in 1756.

However, this stately portal and sloping brick path have already been razed—along with the hideous concrete parking garage—for Bellevue's newest facelift. A new facility for the clinics is being built in front of the towering blood-red brick presence of the Old Bellevue building. So as not to completely eradicate the beauty of this grande dame, a glass atrium will enclose the façade, so that the next generations of Bellevue patients can admire its elegant and forbidding architecture.

⸙

The new lobby of Bellevue—soon to be replaced by an even newer lobby—is a striking semicircular rotunda. This odd-shaped corner of Bellevue was originally a surgical suite. When I was in medical school, it functioned as a repository of "recycled" clothing maintained by the social work department. I recall picking out a pair of serviceable trousers for one of the patients I'd helped as a third-year student. At other times this space was a cafeteria and then a temporary office for administrators. Now it is a bright, high-ceilinged atrium with majestic white columns anchoring into the sleek marble-green floor. When it was converted into the new lobby, the fraying wallpaper was stripped off, revealing a set of frescoes on the curved walls. These turned out to have been a WPA project commissioned in 1941. The broadly outlined figures vaguely echo a socialist-realist style, but the muted acrylic pastels soften the effect. There are women canning fruit in a factory, a couple lugging a heavy wooden cart on a farm, citizens at a town meeting, men lifting steel girders at a construction site, a mother feeding a baby. The last panel, closest to where I enter each morning, depicts a lawn party. A woman in a simply rendered peach gown is singing before a microphone under a pavilion. A string orchestra plays behind her, clad in formal white dinner jackets. Guests with cocktails congregate on the lawn. I've often wondered if the artist was trying to send a message about class struggle or whether he merely had a soft spot for *The Great Gatsby*.

The artist—David Margolis—was still alive when this rotunda was rescued from its institutional servitude, and he was able to touch up the paintings. Apparently he'd been a realist with uncanny foresight: he had covered the original paintings with a layer of wax, just in case they got plastered over at some point.

Margolis was present when the rotunda was the setting for the first poetry/prose reading of the *Bellevue Literary Review*, when more than a hundred people gathered to celebrate the oddly natural presence of literature in the lobby of a city hospital better known for its alcoholics, lunatics, and Riker's prisoners. He mingled with the crowd, periodically stopping in front of the different pictures, as if amazed that his children had survived such a long and tempestuous journey. Shortly before the fourth *BLR* reading, two years later, Margolis died in his sleep. But his paintings echoed in the cavernous room as the authors read their words aloud.

This rotunda, however, will cease to be the elegant gateway to Bellevue once the new building with its postmodern glass atrium opens.

It is still, however, the same walk through Old Bellevue to get to New Bellevue, past the Greek coffee shop with the sonorous counterman and the flying "whiskey downs," past the candy store with its racks of on-call-sustaining candy bars, down the hall past the security guards toward the elevators to the second floor clinic.

The medical clinic, where I spent every Tuesday afternoon as a resident, also had a face-lift. The clinic is a ring of tiny but functional cubicles joined by the long, sunny "bowling alley"—the outer hallway that lines the perimeter of the floor. The rooms have been painted and renovated with new desks and overhead bookshelves. Each room boasts a brand-new computer, as the entire hospital is now entwined in a local network. The exam table is unchanged, however. The brown vinyl covering is scuffed and the legs are rickety, but it is useable. The perennial problem of "wandering" blood pressure cuffs still necessitates the morning ritual of hunting from room to room to snag the appropriately sized variety.

But now I am here as an attending physician. One of those tiny cubicles now has my name permanently affixed to the door—no more scrambling for available rooms, catch-as-catch-can. I rescued a battered file cabinet from the old TB office and dragged it into my room. To cover up the rusty top, I draped it with a vivid blue shawl that I'd purchased in Peru. Museum prints— cheap 8½×11 reproductions of works by David Hockney, Wins-

low Homer, and Matisse, along with an untitled Japanese print
—hang on my wall, the frames drilled into the concrete by the
maintenance men to prevent the drift phenomenon. Already, the
three houseplants I'd brought in to liven up the office have
"drifted," one after the other. I'm considering the plastic type, but
it is unclear if that will prove any less desirable to those who participate in the drifting process.

I suddenly have less need for a white coat. For so many years
my white coat was my portable office. In the pockets I carted
around my stethoscope; reflex hammer; beeper; index cards of
patients; the *Sanford Guide to Antimicrobial Therapy*; the *Facts
and Formulas* book with page 30 folded over for easy access to
the three types of renal tubular acidosis; cheat sheets for cardiac-
arrest protocols and antiarrhythmic drips; the NCEP guidelines
for cholesterol treatment; disposable drug-company pens; EKG
calipers; 20-gauge IV needles; 23-gauge butterfly needles; alcohol
swabs; 4×4 gauze; chewing gum; butterscotch candies; and small
tubes of hand cream to counter the effects of the witheringly dry
air that seems to be present on all hospital wards. Now I have a
real desk. The top drawer even locks! I have disgorged the con-
tents of my white coat into my desk, and now all my tools—those
that I had been trained to rely on—are within arm's reach.

The white coat is somewhat superfluous but still has sentimen-
tal value. It sits parked in my office locker. The insignia on the
breast pocket reads *Attending Physician,* but I wear it only occasionally: when I attend on the wards and need to carry my stethoscope or when it's chilly in the clinic and I've forgotten to bring a
sweater.

Back at Bellevue as an attending. How odd and how wonder-
ful it feels to be back. As though no time and so much time has
passed. The small towns of Florida, New Mexico, and New England were a breather from the clamor of Manhattan. Working in
private practice and small clinics had been so much easier than
negotiating Bellevue—less running around, less bureaucracy, less
sheer physical effort to accomplish small tasks. But I missed the

wild variety of patients, the open-door policy, and the cama-
raderie of being part of a vast network of smart and dry-humored
doctors.

Most important in my time away, though, was the time *not*
practicing medicine. The time traveling through Mexico study-
ing Spanish instead of memorizing the twenty types of vasculitis.
The time spent blissfully lost in the novels of A.B. Yehoshua
and Mario Vargas Llosa in the Peruvian Andes—slowing down
to savor each sentence, rolling the sensual prose over my tongue,
slaking the parching effects of a decade's worth of medical journals, with their sterile passive verbs and cloying anonymous first-
person plural. The time spent chatting with locals and fellow
travelers in the cafés of Oaxaca and Arequipa and learning, in
real time, about the infinite variety of life paths. Learning that
there is, indeed, a route besides the high school–college–medical
school–graduate school–residency trajectory through which one
can traverse life and still be successful. The time spent wandering through the towns of Guatemala seeing where many of my
Bellevue patients had grown up. The time spent slogging through
Spanish translations of *The Wizard of Oz*, appreciating the challenge my patients faced navigating their health care in my English-
speaking world. And the time spent doing nothing, with no
place to be and no one to answer to and no beeper to disturb my
solitude.

All along I knew I would return to Bellevue. As I traveled and
worked, I felt two simultaneous processes at work in my body. I
was airing myself out, digesting the last ten years, but I was also
preparing to go back. Bellevue was the gauge with which I judged
all my clinical experiences on the locum tenens circuit, and my
convictions about returning kept the unsettling rootlessness of
travel at bay. These bookends provided a framework in which to
stretch and experiment. When a faculty position in the medical
clinic opened up, I jumped at it, though I couldn't completely
erase the regrets of giving up the travel-on-a-whim lifestyle.

It's strange to be an attending in this building where I spent ten years as a student and resident. I associate these spacious hallways with always having someone above to answer to or to learn from. The third-year medical students turn to the sub-interns, and the subs depend on the interns. The interns answer to the second-year residents and the second-years rely on the senior residents. The senior residents get advice from the chief residents and the fellows. The chiefs and the fellows are supervised by the attendings.

It's not that I feel that I've finally clawed to the top of the heap and now I can step on everyone else—not at all. Rather, it is the odd sensation of making medical decisions without the requirement, or even the convention, of discussing them with someone else. It is like performing a familiar physical maneuver but not having to flex that muscle you used for so many years. The option of conferring with a colleague remains—the other attendings are friendly, and fully half are Bellevue alumni themselves—but by and large I make all the medical decisions on my own. I choose which antibiotic to use, decide when to commit someone to a lifetime of blood pressure treatment, conclude that a stress test isn't needed. Or I advise the residents in the clinic on these decisions; reassuring them on their judgment, reminding them of other considerations, or intervening to prevent errors. But I, personally, am no longer part of a team, except when I attend on the wards three months each year. Even then, I'm not really part of it; I'm just the supervisor.

Without a team, Bellevue feels much less like the battle trenches. The struggle to keep above water that I'd felt as a medical student and as a resident is strangely absent. I worry less that I am going to kill someone and more about keeping up with the fast-paced schedule. In this sense, being an attending in the Bellevue clinic is far more similar to my locum tenens private practice experiences than it is to my ten years of training in this very same hospital. Working in the clinic is decidedly civilized compared to residency, but of course it has its moments as well: two patients booked for the same time slot, missing charts, Bangladeshi patients without interpreters, and the endless negotiations required to get appointments in less than six months for the cardiology and GI clinics.

8:30 A.M. Doing intakes—interviews with new patients to the clinic. First one is Carola Castaña, a petite thirty-five-year-old Brazilian who immigrated to the United States three months ago. She folds her hands in her lap as I begin to take her history. She understands my questions better if I ask in Spanish rather than English, but her Portuguese replies are Greek to me, so she struggles to answer in English.

Her main complaint is that her joints hurt. Which ones? All of them.

How long? Since age twelve.

Ever see a doctor? Once, as a child. They just told me that I had arthritis and gave me ibuprofen.

No X-rays or blood tests? No.

I start down the long line of questions, but we are stymied by language. I give up and reach for her hands. A principle of internal medicine holds that it's all in the history. An astute clinician should be able to unearth any diagnosis just by asking the right questions. The physical exam is almost an afterthought, a mere confirmation of the already-ascertained diagnosis. But Ms. Castaña silently and unwittingly puts this axiom to shame.

Her history has led me nowhere, but her hands subsume the work of logical reasoning. Her hands are severely ulnar-deviated: the fingers sail off course, angling out to the sides instead of straight forward. They point away from her body as though she is gesturing for the waters to part. The tips crane upward, forming a line of swan necks. The joints that connect her fingers to her hands are swollen like robin's eggs—bulbous, bony protrusions. This young emissary from Brazil has handed me the hands of rheumatoid arthritis, untreated for twenty-three years. These are hands that I have seen only in textbooks.

I explain what she has.

Is there is a cure? she asks.

Cure? I sigh. No.

But there are lots of treatments, I hasten to add. Lots of treatments—this time I say it with more energy in my voice. I wish I possessed diversity in my Spanish so that I could reword my phrases for extra emphasis and depth. But I have only one way to say each thing. If only I'd spent more time in Mexico.

I arrange for X-rays and labs and I give Ms. Castaña a prescription for hydroxychloroquine. Malaria medicines for arthritis—sounds crazy, but it works. I try to explain that in Spanish. At the last minute I remember to add a G6PD assay to the blood tests. Can't give hydroxychloroquine until you check the G6PD. Whew, almost missed that one. G6PD deficiency is not that common in the general population, but it can cause hemolytic anemia with certain medications, and hydroxychloroquine is one of them. Good thing that some facts stick around from residency.

I instruct Ms. Castaña not to take the medicine until I call her tomorrow with the G6PD results. I am glad that she has a phone; I don't take that for granted with my patients. In my head I plan to call the lab today at lunchtime to expedite tests and get the results by this afternoon and then call her before I leave work tonight. Wouldn't it be great if she could start her twenty-three-year-delayed treatment today instead of tomorrow?

9:00 A.M. 54-year-old Dominican woman. Sore throat, back pain. *No, señora, no necesita antibióticos por un virus.* Have you tried exercise for your back? Heating pads are helpful.

9:20 A.M. 37-year-old Bangladeshi man. New-onset diabetes, limited English. Will it be pills or insulin? It's my decision.

9:40 A.M. 41-year-old Mauritanian woman. Dizziness, can't sleep, neck hurts, back hurts, stomach hurts, chest pain. Hmm... underlying depression? Drug use? Domestic violence? Political torture? The diagnostic possibilities are endless.

10:00 A.M. 72-year-old Puerto Rican man. Hypertension, ran out of meds last month. *Señor,* you can't ever let your pills run out. *Es muy importante.* You've got to take those pills every single day, not just when you have a headache. Otherwise you could get a stroke or a heart attack. You can always come to the clinic for a refill—you don't even need an appointment.

10:20 A.M. 63-year-old Ecuadoran woman. Back pain, shoulder pain, foot pain, raising little grandchildren isn't easy at my age. *Señora*, I know. *Es muy difícil.* Is there anyone in the family who can help you? You might try getting shoes without heels. We do have psychologists who speak Spanish. And don't forget about the mammogram; you're way overdue.

Rushing through intakes tenses the muscles of my back, especially the spot just below my right scapula. These intakes are supposed to be screening visits—brief and to the point. The details of the history are supposed to wait until the next visit, but the details are everything and they spill out the minute the door closes behind us and we are alone in my small office. I roll my right shoulder backward to unkink the knot.

Next chart is Yang Qing Xing. I call out the name in the waiting room. No one answers to my probably mangled pronunciation. I seek out the Asians in the room and point to the printed name. They all shake their heads. But somehow, a Mr. Yang is produced from the crowd. He is a tall, lanky man with a face wrinkled far beyond forty-one years. He speaks no English but conveys with his hands that there is someone somewhere who can translate. He hands me a crumpled referral sheet and then I watch him limp awkwardly down the hall to find the communicator who can bridge his life to mine.

The referral is from endocrine clinic and the handwriting, thankfully, is decipherable. *41-year-old Chinese male with papillary carcinoma of the thyroid. Thyroid removed and radioactive iodine treatment given last year. Cancer cured. Needs general medical care.*

I guess it finally occurred to the endocrinologist that Mr. Yang should have an internist to worry about the rest of him now that his cancer is cured. Mr. Yang is a young man—someone has to check his cholesterol and make sure he's up to date with his tetanus shots. While I wait for him to locate his interpreter, I check his labs in the computer. His TSH (thyroid-stimulating hormone) level last month was way off: his thyroxine dose needs to be lowered or even discontinued altogether.

Mr. Yang returns with two young Chinese guys sporting baggy jeans, beepers, ice cream cones, and bottled spring water. Turns out that Mr. Yang speaks only Fukienese, though he can understand a bit of Mandarin. One of the young men speaks Fukienese and Cantonese but little English. The other speaks good English and Mandarin, but no Fukienese. Needless to say, each question takes an endless time to traverse the space between us.

I explain that I will be Mr. Yang's regular doctor, that I will take care of his whole body, not just his thyroid. Mr. Yang conveys that his endocrinologist had told him to stop taking his thyroxine for two weeks (good, the endocrinologist saw that most recent TSH level in the computer). Ever since he stopped taking his pills, though, he's had trouble with his right leg. It just doesn't move well. He wants to restart his medicine.

I ask if he's ever had leg problems before, and he denies any. I ask the question again, not willing to trust just one cycle of translation. One of the young men says that he's translated for Mr. Yang before, at another clinic appointment, and that Mr. Yang didn't have a limp then.

"Common things happen commonly," the saying in medicine goes. Or, "When you hear hooves, think horses, not zebras." I'm sure there is a simple explanation for his limp. What about an old sports injury? I ask. Or plain old arthritis. Maybe he tripped on the bus. Are his shoes too tight?

Mr. Yang shakes his head as each of my questions is processed for him. No, he insists. It all started two weeks ago when the doctor told me to stop taking my thyroxine pills. Just let me start the medicine again, he says, and I will be okay.

I scour my brain: can leg weakness be some bizarre rebound effect of stopping thyroxine? No, that's crazy. The half-life of thyroxine is several weeks; his body probably hasn't even noticed that he's stopped taking the pills.

Somehow, via the circuitous linguistic orbit, the following line from Mr. Yang emerges: "I feel like Christopher Reeve—my head is fine but I can't move my body."

I give up with the questions, realizing that I am not getting anywhere with the history and that time is running quickly. The pile of intake charts is growing and if I don't get a move on it, I will have to work right through lunch. Again.

I skip right to the physical exam.

Mr. Yang places one foot on the step of the exam table but wavers as he tries to pull himself up. The two young men spring to his side and steady him. Their squat muscular arms guide him up to the table and help him swivel his skinny body around into a sitting position. While I listen to Mr. Yang's lungs I recall a patient I saw on my very first day as an attending in the clinic. My first day back at Bellevue. She'd been sent over from Employee Health because her blood sugar was 130; the referral said *Rule out diabetes*. I took a complete history, asking about all aspects of her health. Like every other patient I'd seen that morning, she also complained of back pain. I'd actually palpated her spinal column and even documented in the chart the absence of point tenderness—more than I usually did for back pain. But this was just run-of-the-mill back pain. Try some ibuprofen, I said.

Three days later she was paralyzed. Needed emergency surgery for acute spinal-cord compression—a lymphoma tumor at T7. Surgery, radiation, weeks of rehab. Now she has only a limp, thank God, and manages to walk with a cane.

With her limp in my peripheral vision, I do more than the usual neuro exam on Mr. Yang. Using my rubber hammer I bang not only his knees but also his elbows and ankles. I run through the twelve cranial nerves. I verify sensation of light touch, pain, and vibration—it all seems normal. I even check rectal tone to test the spinal nerves. But when I check flexion and extension of his muscles, his right leg really is weaker than his left.

I can't decide what to do. Do I send him home and see if it gets better in a few days, like most every other ache and pain that I see in the clinic? Or do I need to do a stat X-ray right now? Is there something that I'm missing in his history? I leave the room to get a quick curbside consult with a colleague in the bowling alley. I tell her my story about the lady with a spinal-cord tumor. She doesn't think it sounds like the same thing. But if it'll make you more comfortable, she says, get an X-ray of the spinal column today and then have him come back in two days. See if it's gotten better or worse.

My stomach nags at me. Am I about to miss something big, or am I making a big deal over nothing? Gotta decide quickly—the clerk has just tossed four more charts in the intake bin. The decision is mine, and mine alone. Two vastly different paths could branch out from my decision: I could reassure Mr. Yang that it's nothing and send him home, or I could start calling X-ray and CT and orthopedics and cajole stat evaluations from them—thereby falling even further behind in my work—and make Mr. Yang and his two interpreters—who probably have other places to go—spend hours schlepping around the hospital to do all these tests.

My choice will send him marching down one path or the other. A wince in my right shoulder reminds me of that aching muscle. There's no one hovering above me to whom I can punt the responsibility. There is advice from colleagues, but then I am left with the independence or loneliness—depending on how one looks at it—of my own decision. I can't afford to guess wrong. If only I could speak directly with Mr. Yang to pick up the subtleties of his descriptions and match his body language to his history.

Or, my colleague adds, you could call neuro to come see him; they usually come reasonably quickly. But don't bother trying to call endocrine; they won't call you back until a week from Tuesday.

I call the neurology consult, who says he can swing by in forty-five minutes. I am impressed and thankful. I park the polyglot trio in the room next door and set about catching up on the stack of charts that is now spilling out of the intake bin.

My next patient is an elderly Egyptian woman from Alexandria. She screws up her mouth. "I here since eight thirty! Is it because I am new patient? Because my English is no good?"

No, I promise her. You know how things are in the clinic. I

catch her eye and hope she smiles back sympathetically. But we'll take care of your diabetes, don't you worry. Her face relaxes a little bit. When's the last time you've had a mammogram, Mrs. Jamila? Never? Well, it's time.

11:00 A.M. 59-year-old Puerto Rican man with emphysema. Had another attack last week. *Señor, necesite dejar de fumar!* You can't smoke if you have emphysema. And you have to get your flu shot every year, *por favor*. No, the vaccine won't make you sick, I promise. I get the shot every year and I never get sick. *Nunca!*

11:15 A.M. 33-year-old white man with schizophrenia. Used to be a computer programmer before he had his first psychotic break. Now he's in a halfway house and able to take care of the basics in his life on his current medications. Needs a physical exam to get his benefits. Are you in touch with your family at all? No? Is there anyone at all you can turn to?

11:30 A.M. The neuro consult knocks on my door. He has just finished examining Mr. Yang.

"Good call," he says with admiration. "You just picked up a brain tumor."

Brain tumor? The pinch under my scapula suddenly ratchets like a drill deep into my back. The consult leads me back to Mr. Yang. He demonstrates the subtle hyperreflexia of the right leg, the pronator drift of his right arm. Mr. Yang's face is carved with wrinkles, maybe from years of laboring in the sun. I can't read the expression among the deeply etched corrugations. How much, I wonder, has been translated back to him through the serpentine linguistic channels? Still dazed, I fill out the hospital admission forms, and the neuro guy whisks Mr. Yang off for an emergent CT scan before I can gather my thoughts. I wish I knew how to say "Good luck" in Fukienese. Or "I'm so sorry."

11:45 A.M. 61-year-old black male. Arthritis in the knees. Exercise the muscles. Take the ibuprofen with food, otherwise your stomach will hurt.

12:00 noon. 32-year-old Dominican woman. Heartburn. Deaf

patient. Sign language interpreter is stuck in pediatrics. That's okay, we'll just print on paper. Luckily she can read English. *TAKE THIS PILL TWICE A DAY*, I write in block letters, careful to keep it legible. *IT WILL MAKE YOUR STOMACH FEEL BETTER.*

12:30. All the intakes are done. Finally. Grab my cheese sandwich and start preparing for the afternoon. There's a third-year medical student coming to my clinic this afternoon. Our topic today is evidence-based medicine. I rifle through my files, hunting for an article that demonstrates those academic principles while still being relevant to clinical practice.

1:00 P.M. Explaining evidence-based medicine to the third-year medical student. She sits stiffly on the chair with her white jacket buttoned up and her *Washington Manual of Medicine* sliding over the edge of her pocket. She nods mechanically at each thing I say, even when I ask if she has any questions. Did I look this nervous when I was a third-year?

I leaf through the paper on coronary disease with her, pointing out the differences between primary versus secondary prevention of heart attacks and how not to be fooled by the *relative* risk reductions quoted in the study. You have to go by the *absolute* risk reduction. She is still nodding mechanically. I pause from my explanations. Have you ever even seen a patient with a heart attack? I ask. She shakes her head no. I flip the paper over and start drawing a simple diagram of the heart with its coronary arteries. Got to start with the basics.

2:00 P.M. 64-year-old Puerto Rican woman with hypertension who hasn't had a pelvic exam in decades. Elijida Rivera hates the GYN clinic. I don't blame her; I spent time in that clinic as a medical student and it reminded me of cattle being herded through a factory. But she will allow the Pap smear in the medicine clinic. I am reminded of the young Navajo woman with acne and I am again honored that a patient would trust me with this most intimate of examinations.

I lug the exam table from the wall to free up the leg rests. It heaves forward in fits and starts, and I feel that spot under my right scapula strain. I jam a tongue depressor in the arm of the lamp so it won't float up to the ceiling. I lay out my equipment on a clean paper towel spread on top of the industrial garbage pail. I print her information on all three lab forms, and I stamp labels for the specimens. I hold the speculum steady with my left hand while my nondominant right hand is forced to take the samples, spread them on the slide, spray the fixative. My kingdom for a nurse like Karen. But my Spanish is adequate to explain most of what I'm doing. Glad I spent that extra week in Peru working on the imperative.

3:00 P.M. The neuro consult drops by. Not one, but four! Four big goobers in Mr. Yang's brain, he says. They'll give steroids and radiation to shrink the swelling. That will improve his symptoms, but the neurosurgeons won't operate if there are already four intracranial masses. Six months to a year, they say…

I close my eyes for a moment and I see Mr. Yang's wrinkled face with the expression that I can't read and can't match with his words. And what did he make of *my* facial expressions that he couldn't match with *my* words? I am suddenly overwhelmed by the fear and loneliness that I imagine he will feel, upstairs in a hospital bed, maybe for weeks, unable to communicate with anyone except when the Fukienese interpreter is available.

4:30 P.M. I check Ms. Castaña's labs. No G6PD results to be found. I call the lab and they tell me there was no order for one. But I know I checked it off on the requisition slip. No dice, they say, we don't have a requisition for it. Damn! I don't want to make Ms. Castaña come back again for another blood draw. Twenty-three years of inappropriate treatment is long enough. I want to show her that we'll do it right this time. That we'll take care of her at Bellevue. That she'll get care as good and as prompt as she would at any private practice.

I wish I could do something for Mr. Yang. Something that could change his prognosis. But he has been whisked away from me. Whisked away on a stretcher by the neuro consult, whisked away by the language barrier that reduces the doctor-patient relationship to its most crassly bare bones, whisked away by his disease that we had assumed was cured. *Harrison's* says that papillary cancer of the thyroid—the type that Mr. Yang has—rarely metastasizes; that *follicular* cancer is the one to worry about. I remember memorizing that one for the boards. Another patient unwittingly disproving the rules. The least I can do is expedite Ms. Castaña's treatment. I just need that damn G6PD.

Residency was only a few years ago; I still know the back channels. I call Central Accession and track down the sample number. I dial hematology and ask if there is any blood left over from her CBC to send to the special hematology lab for a G6PD. The tech is cranky: "There are a thousand samples; call back in an hour."

6:00 P.M. Finally home. Got to leave for Spanish class in a half hour. Spanish is my lingua franca in this clinic. I telephone hematology while I stuff *Gramática Española Avanzada* in my bag. The evening-shift tech is much more pleasant. She's able to locate the specimen. And there's enough left over! Just bring over a lab slip, she says kindly, and I'll pop it right in the machine. But I'm home already, I can't bring over a lab slip.

Evening clinic. Who's doing evening clinic tonight? Elaine's got Tuesday nights. Maybe she can walk the lab slip over to the lab.

I call the clinic and talk to the clerk at the front desk, who puts me on hold. I pour a bowl of raisin bran while I'm waiting, trying to keep my crunch away from the phone. Still on hold, I finish my cereal. Where the heck is she? I wash the bowl, keeping the phone cramped between my ear and my neck. That spot behind my right shoulder is acting up. Still on hold. I've got to leave for class, where is she? Finally she returns, informing me that she was finally able to locate the chart in the chart room.

I slap my hand on my forehead, too dumbfounded and annoyed to speak. We don't need the *chart* to get a lab slip, I want to scream.

How could you waste so much precious time? But it's not worthwhile to yell at the clerks. It never accomplishes anything and they'll never do you any favors ever again. Gritting my teeth to modulate my voice, I ask her to please connect me to Dr. Feingold's office.

6:15 P.M. I give Elaine the patient's name, the medical record number, the sample number, the name of the tech who approved the add-on test, and which test to order. She fills out the form then transfers me back to the clerk so I can tell the clerk what to do, but there's no answer. And no answer. And no answer.

Fifteen minutes I keep dialing. No answer. Where is the clerk? Where is anybody? I don't know the direct number to Elaine's office and can only phone the front desk. Over and over I call, hunting in my fridge for a snack to bring to the three-hour class. At least there's a redial button on my phone. I finally dial the page operator and have Elaine paged overhead. No answer. No one ever hears those overhead pages anyway; it's a total waste of time.

It's 6:30, and I've got to get going. I can't miss Spanish class—tonight we're doing the preterit and the imperfect. I need those tenses. I start randomly calling every desk in the clinic, hoping someone will pick up. After ten calls and many pleas, someone has a heart and connects me to Elaine's office. I am panting with relief.

"Oh," says Elaine, "the clerk walked the lab slip over to the outpatient lab but it was closed."

Of course the second-floor outpatient lab was closed, I want to scream. It's after five P.M. You have to take it to the *fourth-floor* central lab! I slam a Granny Smith apple in my bag. Doesn't anyone know the system around here?

Please, Elaine, could you please drop it off on your way out? Would you mind, please? She hesitates. It's been a long day. "Could I bring it to the lab tomorrow morning on my way in?" she asks.

Nothing personal, but I hate to trust anyone to remember anything. Please, please could you bring it over tonight? It's only two floors up. And there's never any wait for the elevators at this time of day.

Mr. Yang is probably sitting all by himself in his hospital bed. The nurse's evaluation is brief because she can't explain about the daily routine of the ward or ask him if he has any dietary preferences for his meal tray. The interpreters have probably gone home for the day. All the nurse can do is take his blood pressure and pulse. I want it to be right for Ms. Castaña. I want to be able to call her tomorrow with the results like I'd promised. Just because we're a city clinic doesn't mean we can't give our patients medical care like they get in New England or in Florida. I want to live up to my word.

6:45 P.M. Forty-five minutes working on this stupid lab slip. I could've gone back to Bellevue myself and walked it over. Elaine finally agrees. I dash off to Spanish class on my bike.

10:30 P.M. Home. Head still swimming with the preterit tense, I call the lab and track down the heme lady. She's pleasant and helpful. The lab slip was received! Thank you, Elaine, thank you. The tech carried the sample herself to the special hematology section. The G6PD will be done first thing in the morning. Of course I would have liked to have it done tonight, but I'm happy that it will get done at all without making Ms. Castaña come back for another blood draw. Thank you, oh anonymous technician, for getting it done.

I hope.

11:30 P.M. Bed. A few pages of a novel before collapsing under the covers, as the images and people of today swirl in my head, pounding my consciousness. In less than twenty-four hours, my life has swooped into the lives of people of different sizes, shapes, colors, nationalities, and religions. We're more alike than we are different, but the sheer randomness and devastating consequences of illness terrify me. Why them and not me?

My gastrocnemius and soleus muscles effortlessly allow me to bicycle to my Spanish class, while Mr. Yang limps from his tumor. My joints glide smoothly while Carola Castaña's chafe bone against bone. I live in a culture in which medicine is so easily obtainable, yet Carola's arthritis has gone untreated for so many years.

It pains me that there is nothing I can do for Mr. Yang. And that I lack the language skills to offer even the slightest balm of comforting words. Perhaps that is what is driving my obsession with Carola Castaña's arthritis treatment. It is obvious that a one-day delay, after twenty-three years of inadequate treatment, is meaningless. Yet it has consumed my energy. I have spotted one tiny brick in the chaotic rubble that I can attempt to right.

The harrowing state of humanity can be chilling, and if I meditate too long upon it, the ache under my right shoulder bores its way though to my insides. I grab a heating pad, cram it under my shoulder, and crank it to the highest setting. The heat seeps in slowly and I can feel my brain gradually easing its frenetic grip on awakeness.

Yes, the world is random and cruel. And yes, there is not much an individual can do to alter that.

But maybe re-righting one brick will provide a scrap of order to the chaos, a sliver of support for a future column. Maybe Carola will finally get her medications. Maybe that is cause enough for joy.

Tomorrow: Another day at the Bellevue clinic.

My eyelids give up fighting and finally sink, closed.

CHAPTER FIVE

THE JOURNEY

THE FIRST GATE CREAKED OPEN and I stepped into the anteroom where the sand-filled bins for unloading ammunition sat like ungainly marsupials. All guns and bullets had to be submitted, separately, to the glass-enclosed guard before entering the prison ward.

"He's all ready to go," the intern had told me earlier that morning. "His diabetes is tuned, his congestive heart failure is stable. His blood pressure's controlled and there's only moderate renal insufficiency. We'll ship him back to Riker's and they can follow his blood sugar at their infirmary. You just have to sign his chart." She'd flipped her stethoscope into a curl and neatly slid it back into the pocket of her white coat. "I mean, he's still complaining of pain anywhere you touch him, but he probably has a bit of diabetic neuropathy pain. Personally, I think it's the hyper-pain thing all those cocaine addicts have."

I had nodded my head as she spoke, scanning the list of thirty-two patients I had to learn on my first day as the ward attending this month. "Right," I'd said to her. "The hyper-pain thing."

After three more metal gates heaved open, I strode to the final gate, the one that actually led to the ward. The one that actually had to be opened by a human with an actual key. "Gate, please," I hollered to the empty space, with the appropriate amount of annoyance in my voice. Through the widely spaced, crosshatched bars of the gate, I could see the edge of the battered security desk. A chair scraped, and a paunchy officer ambled around the corner with an ancient skeleton key gripped in his fist—the massive iron type of key you might imagine in a Dickens novel. He rattled the key in the lock and the door swung open toward me like an old-fashioned gate on a farm. The arc was wide and almost playful. I was tempted to grab on and ride the bars during their pendulous swing out into the hallway, like a rancher in a moment of conviviality with her steers. But that wouldn't have been seemly.

The patient rooms were spread along one side of the hall of the prison ward—three beds and a bathroom in each one. Expansive internal windows provided the nurses and the officers and the clerks and the dietary aides and anyone else walking by with a full view of the patients' rooms. The bathroom was closest to the window in each room, equipped with stainless-steel toilets and sinks. No porcelain like the rest of the patients in the hospital. A concrete wall, however, rose three discreet feet from the floor, so that the lower halves of the prisoners' bodies were obscured from view when they used the facilities.

At the far end of each room was the real window facing outside. A real estate agent's dream was available free of charge: panoramic river views, unobscured Manhattan skyline, vast southern exposure. But the windows were cut off by a thick metal mesh. The interlocking grid of metal was so tightly laced that a probing finger could not touch the actual glass. The flood of sun was diffused into multitudes of puny rays whose sum of intensity could never equal the whole. But the window mesh was painted a pale yellowish-white, as was the rest of the ward, in a laudable effort to soften the setting.

"Mr. McCreary?" I asked, approaching a lump huddled under the sheets in room 19-South-33A. The lump rolled slowly toward me and the sheets pulled away from his face. His pasty dark skin was hunched into heavy wrinkles. Whitish-gray hair lay in grizzled clumps around his face.

Mr. McCreary squinted at me in the fading light. How many white coats had paraded by his bedside already? "When am I going to feel better, Doc?" he asked in a soft, gravelly voice before

I could even introduce myself. "It hurts everywhere, specially my legs."

I reached for the sheet but he jumped upright. "No, no," he said, his voice suddenly louder. "You can't touch it. It hurts too much."

I pulled my hand back. "Sorry. Would it be okay if I just looked? No touching, I promise." I marveled at the irony of a convicted felon intimidated by a 5'3" female doctor. How did he handle himself in prison?

He stared at me, pondering, then let out a long breath. "You can look," he said, his voice calmer now, "but just don't touch. It's like they's on fire. All those damn doctors been touching my legs, poking and prodding every day, and nothing gets any better."

I folded back the sheet, wondering who *he* might have intimidated before robbing or raping or shooting them. What crime had landed him in prison? But you weren't supposed to ask. Those were the rules.

Underneath were just two ordinary skinny legs—no ulcers from diabetes or track marks from drug injection. A few bruises from a lifetime of use, but normal-looking legs, pulled up toward Mr. McCreary's chest in a protective position.

Friends often ask me what it's like to take care of criminals. They're just regular patients, I always tell them, and I tried to believe that. In fact, most of the prisoners we treated had been involved in petty crime or small drug deals. Many were barely older than kids and were quite respectful of the doctors. But I remember hearing about one guy who had murdered someone over five dollars.

"I'm just going to check your pulse," I said, lowering my fingertips to the top of his right foot and letting them rest gently between the tendons of the first and second toes.

"Yee-ow!" he cried out, as though I'd just pierced him with an 18-gauge IV. "You're killing me. Jeez."

"From what I can see," I said, "it looks like you have diabetic neuropathy. After many years of having diabetes, it can affect the nerves in the feet and make them feel numb or like pins and needles."

"Well, I never had no diabetes for years."

No diabetes for years? I suddenly felt a little off balance. How could he not know that he had diabetes? Wasn't that my whole case for explaining to him the permanency of the situation? "You, uh, didn't have diabetes?"

"Well, everybody been saying diabetes this and diabetes that round here, but this all is news to me."

"Didn't your doctor at home ever say you had diabetes?" My mind floated back to Mr. McCreary's chart, which I'd reviewed earlier, with its sky-high glucose values and documentation of every known complication of long-standing diabetes.

"I don't remember. Maybe someone said something or other 'bout my sugar, but no one never said nothing 'bout no diabetes. Besides, I ain't seen no doctor in some while." He shrugged, his neck sinking into his skinny shoulders. "Doc, listen. When am I going to feel better?"

"Diabetic neuropathy is not one of those things that gets cured overnight. It's a long-term thing and it's not the kind of thing you have to stay in the hospital for." Decreasing length-of-stay was the mantra hammered into our heads by our administrators.

"I don't care what you gotta do. I just want to feel better. You can't kick me out when I'm hurting like this."

"I know it's painful, but diabetic neuropathy is something we treat as an outpatient. We'll send you back with some pain medicines, and then the doctors in the infirmary can adjust the dose."

"Send me back? Back where?"

"Riker's. Where you came from."

"Riker's?" He pulled himself up in the bed. "I'm going to Riker's?"

Whoops. Did I reveal something I wasn't supposed to? You weren't ever supposed to tell prisoners when they were going to be discharged, but I wasn't talking specific dates, I was just talking about what would happen once he got there. "Isn't that where you came from?"

"I didn't come from no Riker's," he said, now sitting upright. "No?"

"They just arrested me last week, up in the Bronx, and then I ended up here. Am I going to Riker's?"

I didn't have the foggiest idea. The details of the criminal justice system were murky to me. I knew there was the Precinct, Central Booking, Riker's Island, the Tombs, and a few other links in the chain, but I didn't know the order or relation of any of them. "Well, wherever you go," I fumbled, trying to get back on the medical track, "you'll get follow-up care to adjust your medicines." Had I just told a bald-faced lie, or was I merely overly optimistic about the synergy of the medical and criminal justice systems? But that was what *should* happen, right? We'd start his medical care, but then he'd follow up as an outpatient wherever he ended up.

The nurse wheeled his cart in and handed Mr. McCreary a paper cup with his afternoon meds.

"All these pills," he grumbled. "A man can't live with all these pills." He cocked his head back and the pills clattered faintly against each other as they slid down his throat.

"Mr. McCreary," I said. "I know these pills are annoying, but they are important. You have to control your diabetes and your blood pressure."

"Listen, Doc. Just tell me when I'm going to feel better." He crushed the empty paper cup in his hand. "You know I wasn't always like this. I used to play football. I used to do construction work. I used to really get around. When am I going to get better?"

I slumped back against the pale yellow concrete wall. Through the small holes in the wire mesh over the far window I could make out the glistening East River. It was dispersed in little bits, like a pointillist painting. The intern was right—Mr. McCreary *was* suffering from the hyper-pain thing. But it wasn't from his cocaine.

Mr. McCreary was crossing the river, and not the one that separated Manhattan from Queens and Riker's Island. He was crossing the river that separated the healthy from the sick. He was emigrating from the land of insouciant good health over to the land of disease with a one-way ticket.

Mr. McCreary had somehow managed to stay ignorant of, or oblivious to, the insidious progression of his diabetes over the years. Most people learn their diagnoses early on, when symptoms are typically mild. They grow accustomed to the pills and the blood tests and the doctors' visits. They have time to acclimate themselves to their illnesses. They are able to break them in, like new shoes.

But not Mr. McCreary. He was going cold turkey from the healthy to the sick. All at once he was discovering that he had diabetes and hypertension. And heart disease and kidney problems. That his diabetes would cause burning pains in his feet that would probably never go away completely. That he might never be able to play football again. That he might become insulin-dependent, impotent, amputated, in a wheelchair. That his heart could give out. I couldn't even bear to mention that his moderate renal insufficiency was just the first step along that yellow-brick road toward lifelong hemodialysis.

Mr. McCreary had hyper-pain, all right, and his pain was genuine. He had the pain of being forced by his diabetes to say good-bye to the man he was. And he had to do it here in the dim halls of the Bellevue prison ward, not even knowing where he would be shipped after his discharge. I couldn't even offer him the comfort of the "doctor and patient as team." I couldn't tell him that we could work together to get him on the right regimen of medicines. That we could do everything possible to control his pain. That I would not abandon him as he sailed across that painful river into the unknown. No, none of that was available for his journey.

I turned back from the East River to Mr. McCreary. What could I say? "Those little capsules you took," I said, "they are for your foot pain. Your doctors, wherever you go, will increase the dose until your pain starts to ease. And if they don't work, there are other pills to try."

"But when will I get better?" he asked again, this time more insistently.

Some patients never let you off the hook.

"Diabetes," I said softly, "is one of those things you can't cure. There are lots of treatments, but no cures."

"You can't send me out like this. You gotta make me better."

You're right, I thought, I *can't* send you out like this, with all this pain. I'm a doctor—I'm *supposed* to make you feel better. But how can I explain that it's just not possible? "I wish I had the magic pill," I said, "but it doesn't exist. It's going to be a day-by-day thing."

"I don't care about no diabetes. I just want to get better. You can't send me out feeling like this." He sank back down in bed, seeming to melt into the sheets.

I looked back to the pointillist view of the East River. C'mon, coward, tell him the truth. Tell him he's not going to get better and he'll probably have a lifetime of pain. You know the stats—he'll be on dialysis in a year, his sight will deteriorate, he'll be taking pills and injections round the clock, and he'll likely be dead from a heart attack long before he's eligible for parole.

From the window I could see all the way to the other side of the water. For me, the other side was just Queens—factories and row houses. For him, the other side was illness and death. I was suddenly stuck by the awe of the moment. Because most people are absorbed so gradually by their disease, it is rare to be suspended in this exact moment of transition. I felt like I was watching a movie that had been paused at the climax. Mr. McCreary's years of denial or ignorance allowed him to be frozen in this moment. I imagined that other doctors before me had tried to convince him of the seriousness of his illness, or maybe he had truly avoided the medical system and managed to ignore his symptoms. In either case, it was at this moment that he was being confronted by the gale force of illness.

How long could the flimsy twigs of his denial hold out? I assumed they were flimsy because the reality of chronic pain and hemodialysis and amputations would eventually knock down any denial. But maybe not. Maybe even those harsh doses of reality could be ignored. The truth was, however, that his illness was forcing him along this journey, denial or no denial.

The paunchy corrections officer poked his head in. "Doc, you almost done with McCreary? We got some stuff to do with him."

I looked back to the man huddled under the sheets. The beseeching, bewildered look was still on his face.

"I guess I'm about done." I held out my hand to Mr. McCreary, but he didn't take it. "It was nice meeting you. We'll talk some more about this tomorrow."

When I rounded the next morning, Mr. McCreary was gone. "They finally shipped him back," the intern said, the relief palpable in her voice. "Those hyper-pain guys drive you crazy; nothing ever makes them feel better."

I could only nod. "It's a long journey he's got."

"Whaddya mean?" she said. "He'll be at Riker's in time for lunch."

CHAPTER SIX

TORMENT

I GROAN WHEN I CATCH SIGHT of her name on the patient roster. Nazma Uddin. Not again! She is in my clinic office almost every month. I dread her visits, and today is no exception. A small, plump woman, Mrs. Uddin is cloaked in robe, headscarf, and veil, all opaque blue polyester. Only her eyes peer out from the sea of dark blue. She is trailed, as usual, by her eleven-year-old daughter, Azina, who wears a light green gown with a flowered headscarf pinned under her chin but no veil covering her solemn, bespectacled face.

Mrs. Uddin flops into the chair next to my desk with a postural sprawl that is almost teenagerly. Azina perches on the exam table, her white Nikes peeking out from under the full-length gown. Mrs. Uddin unsnaps her veil—something she does only with her female doctor—revealing her weathered cheeks, and the litany begins. "Oh, Doctor," she says, pinching the sides of her head with skin-paling force, "the pain is no good." After this brief foray into English, she slips into Bengali, aiming her barrage of complaints at Azina, who translates them to me in spurts while fiddling with her wire-rimmed glasses. There is abdominal pain and headache, diarrhea and insomnia, back pain and aching arches, a rash and gas pains, itchy ears and a cough, no appetite. And more headache.

The feeling begins: a dull cringing in my stomach that gradually creeps outward, until my entire body is sapped by foreboding and dread. I feel myself slipping into her morass, and the smothering sensation overcomes me. If she doesn't stop, I will drown in her complaints.

I fight it, but it is impossible. I know that I should be focused on Mrs. Uddin's words, but I fear for my sanity and my ability to get through this visit and move on to the next ten patients.

And so I begin to filter. I begin to ignore a certain percentage of what is being said, nodding vaguely, murmuring offhandedly—shortcuts to suggest I am engaged but are merely smoke screens to keep her at bay. I scan the computer while she moans about her shins and her coccyx, and I see that she has been to neurology clinic, rehab clinic, pain management clinic, gynecology clinic, podiatry clinic, GI clinic... all in the five weeks since I last saw her.

"Doctor," she is pleading with me, now in English, and I hurriedly refocus on her. "Why so much pain?" The leathery grain of Mrs. Uddin's skin and her seemingly permanent submersion in the world of the sick make me think of her as elderly. I am always shocked when the computer reminds me that she is thirty-five. "Why, Doctor, why?" Her laments are punctuated by the resonant thud of Azina's sneakers banging repetitively and absentmindedly against the metal exam table.

When not translating, Azina gazes at the posters on the walls. Her eyes drift over to my desk, with its piles of papers, journals, memos, and prescriptions. Our eyes accidentally meet, but her expression is mute, and mine is likely frustrated. Azina turns quickly away and begins fingering the crinkly white paper covering the exam table.

I desperately want to get Mrs. Uddin out of my office. I hate my visits with her, and it is increasingly difficult to mask that. Like all the other doctors who see Nazma Uddin, I'm anxious to write a few more referrals or a few more prescriptions just to get her out of my hair.

The truth is, I can't *do* anything for Mrs. Uddin. I've talked to her endlessly about stress and depression, which I am sure underlie many of her pains, but she never follows through with the psychiatry referrals or antidepressant prescriptions. Her resistance to my efforts sometimes makes me feel as though she is in a personal battle against me.

I start to resent her, to hate her, to hate everything about her. I hate to see her name on the roster. I hate to see her in the waiting room. I hate the whine in her voice that is detectable even when she is speaking Bengali. I hate the veil that she wears. Any last bit of cultural sensitivity I possess is washed away. I begin to resent her for her culture. How can she let herself be hidden away in a sea of horrid polyester? How can she buy in to a culture that finds every aspect of her so repulsive or so threatening that it must submerge her in the darkest, most stultifying of material? There is not one iota of design or pattern. No, her body doesn't even merit the slightest print, flower, or delicate fold. Only harsh, opaque, heavy, airless, unforgiving material.

I hate that she routinely keeps her daughter out of school to facilitate her wild overuse of the medical system.

And I hate how she makes me feel so utterly useless.

Whenever I treat one complaint, another bursts to the surface, like a mocking Hydra head: An antacid temporarily relieves her stomach pains, but then she will have palpitations. A migraine medication partially assuages her headache, but then she will have intractable hiccups and swollen knees.

I can't breathe, she says. I don't eat. I don't sleep.

Well, if that's truly the case, I want to retort, how is it that you are still alive?

I stop listening to what she says. I stop believing what she tells me about her symptoms. Stop it, I want to yell at her. Just stop complaining. Go away. Stop bothering me. *You* know and *I* know that this is hopeless.

I shudder as I realize that I am slipping too far. The annoyance and resentment are getting the better of me. But sometimes I wish she would just disappear—out of my office, out of my hospital, out of this city, off this planet. How is it that she emigrated thousands of miles from her obscure village in Bangladesh to end up precisely in the catchment area of my clinic, then randomly in *my* office, when there are a hundred and fifty other medical attendings and residents she could have been assigned to?

Why, I plead with myself, can't I unearth some grain of humanity? Why can't I put my feelings aside to help a patient in need, no matter how annoying?

Back at our first visit—if I can even remember that far—I was probably compassionate. I'm sure I asked open-ended questions and responded with concern to each of her problems.

Now I am the model of the curt, hyperefficient doctor. I ask as few questions as possible for fear of eliciting new, unsolvable complaints. I avoid eye contact. I focus on the computer, tuning out her words, as I copy from my previous note: *Multiple somatic complaints, noncompliant with recommendations for psychiatric therapy*.

I have tried to prioritize her complaints. I have tried setting modest, attainable goals. I have tried to reassure her of her basic good health. I have tried to placate her by ordering every test she requests. I have tried to set limits by refusing to order the tests she requests. I have tried to help her see the connection between stress and symptoms. Nothing helps.

And now I am angry.

"You are healthy," I say to Mrs. Uddin sternly. No reaction.

I turn to the daughter, antagonism rising in my voice. "Tell your mother that she is healthy, that all her tests are normal, that most of these symptoms are related to depression, and that she needs to see the psychiatrist." Azina's face is blank as she translates.

After speaking, the daughter looks down at her sneakers, her light veil tumbling over her shoulders as she lowers her gaze. "Are you almost finished?" she asks.

It takes me a moment to realize that Azina is talking to me. This is the first time Azina has ever addressed me directly.

She looks up at me. "I have to take her home on the bus, and then I have to take another bus to school. I don't want to miss the whole day."

"Can't your mother come to clinic by herself?" I ask, a bit less testily. "We do have interpreters available."

"My mother is afraid to go out by herself," Azina says in a voice that wants to be belligerent but is too weary. "My brother is in college and my father works, so I have to take her to the doctor." She stares back down at her sneakers, which have stopped banging and are now wriggling from side to side like lively caterpillars.

I turn from the computer for a moment and really look at Azina. Her eyes are smooth sandalwood, magnified into iridescent disks by the thick lenses of her glasses. "What is it like at home?" I ask quietly.

This is the first time I've ever addressed Azina as anything other than her mother's mouthpiece. This is the first time I have ever really noticed her.

"She doesn't *do* anything," Azina mumbles. "She just sits there." Azina's face has a prepubescent chubbiness that is somehow incongruous with the seriousness of her headscarf and glasses.

I turn in my chair to face her directly. Tears begin to slide down her cheeks, and her voice rises in a warble. "She doesn't say anything to us. She doesn't cook dinner anymore. She doesn't go anywhere."

My mind begins to paint a picture of the Uddin home, and I see a little girl cut off from her mother, reeling in the wretched vacuum that depression creates—a child conscripted to be the fulcrum of cultures, illnesses, and torments, all while trying to complete fifth grade. I am mortified now that I was so consumed with my own feelings of being overwhelmed when before me sits a child who is drowning—a child grasping the rickety timbers that can barely support her mother and that threaten to sink them both.

It is the innocence of this pain, its simplicity, that both shocks me back to reality and humbles me. I realize that never, in all my visits with Mrs. Uddin, have I paid any attention to Azina; she was always a mere appendage to her mother's appointments, trailing along, obediently translating and directing, as so many first-generation children do.

In medicine we always seek objective data to confirm a diagnosis, something that is often tricky with "difficult" patients. But Azina *is* the objective data, the stark evidence of the magnitude of my patient's pain. Though I'd like to write off Mrs. Uddin as just another complainer, as one who can't hiccup without demanding an MRI, she is truly suffering. Her daughter is truly suffering.

I am not suffering.

I am actually the complainer. I'm the one who can't face this patient without immediately rolling my eyes and turning off my compassion. The reality is that I am profoundly discomfited by my inability to treat Mrs. Uddin, and she is simply the thorn that continually reminds me how limited my skills can be.

Though physicians inquire about patients' social history as part of the full medical interview, it is usually given only lip service. We tend to view our patients as just that: patients. They exist only in our office, on our wards, in our clinics. We forget that 99 percent of their lives are lived—or suffered—without us. We often react as though their illness is a personal battle between doctor and patient, when, in fact, we doctors are bit players. The real battle is between the patient and his or her world: spouses, children, work, community, daily activities. It is within this grander tapestry that the threads and snags of bodily dysfunction introduce rents in the fabric, even wholesale unraveling. It is often only when we are allowed to glimpse the greater weave of our patients' existence that we can truly understand what illness is.

I take the hands of both Azina and her mother, for they are both my patients now. "Depression is a painful illness," I say. "Broken souls hurt as much as broken bones, and the pain spreads to everyone around them." I explain about antidepressant medications and the importance of psychotherapy, and we negotiate a contract for treatment. This time, I include a stipulation that Mrs. Uddin come alone or with her husband, that Azina must stay in school.

Azina wipes her tears. Mrs. Uddin gathers her papers and snaps the veil back over her face. She promises to take the medications and see the psychiatrist.

Of course, we have been down this road many times before, and I won't be surprised if she's back next month with a new physical ailment, not taking her antidepressants, having missed the appointment with the psychiatrist. And I won't be surprised if I, again, dread the visit.

But I think, or at least I hope, that I will no longer view Nazma Uddin as a personal torment. Azina has cured me of that.

CHAPTER SEVEN

VISION

TODAY IS THE BEGINNING OF ANOTHER new month attending on the wards. I've had to meet thirty-nine new patients on 16-West. December is always a busy month on the wards; pneumonia and flu are rampant and the cold weather drives many of the homeless and the fragile to the hospital. Mr. Karlin was the fourteenth patient on my list. When I asked my routine "How are you doing?" he methodically pushed his bedside tray away from the bed, eyed me for a long moment, and then gathered his breath.

"This hospital is abysmal! No one ever comes when I press the call button. I barely see the doctors. The food is pitiful. There is so much noise that I can never sleep. My reading glasses got lost in the ambulance, so I can't read. But that doesn't matter since my bed light doesn't work. But *that* doesn't matter because no one's given me my glaucoma drops since I got to this hospital, so I can't see a damn thing anyway!

"I can shout for hours about my pain and I may as well be in the Serengeti for all the response I get. My roommate is a yowling loony. They come stab you for blood at four o'clock in the morning. I haven't moved my bowels in nearly a week. The physical therapist is a prima donna."

He stopped abruptly and squinted at my ID card. "And which kind of doctor did you say you were?"

Mr. Karlin was a seventy-five-year-old white man, admitted to Bellevue two weeks ago after passing out in his apartment—syncope, in medical terminology. He'd been caught between the sink and the bathtub for two days, unable to extricate himself; the land-lord had to break down the door to get him out.

A white scruff of beard covered Mr. Karlin's face, giving him a Hemingway-type look, but his sunken eyes and sallow cheeks bespoke more soul-battering illness than testosterone-charged bravado. His hospital course had been complicated by fevers, pneumonia, fluid on the lungs, severe constipation, conjunctivitis, and multiple diagnostic dilemmas. The team told me that he been refusing many of the tests they'd ordered, particularly the ones that made him claustrophobic, which made it impossible to com-plete the medical workup for syncope and all his other conditions.

Mr. Karlin was about as unhappy as a patient could be. I'd been hoping to get away with a few minutes of pleasantries and a brief medical exam so that I could meet all my new patients before lunch then spend the afternoon poring over charts and review-ing the cases with the house staff. But I could see that this was a potential Pandora's box. Obviously, I wasn't going to be able to undo two weeks' worth of complaints in just a few minutes, but if I brushed off his issues in an effort to stay on schedule, I'd quickly end up as just another doctor for him to get annoyed at, something that would do neither of us any good. I needed to make him my ally, but it was not a particularly pleasant experience to be on the receiving end of a tirade of complaints, especially when I hadn't been part of, or even present for, all the bad things that had transpired.

I knew that I needed to gain some credibility with Mr. Karlin in order to break through this impasse. To do that, I needed to solve at least one of his problems, definitively and expeditiously, with-out falling hopelessly behind on my rounds. I also needed to gain credibility with the house staff, to show that I could help relieve some of the more nettlesome problems on their service without infringing on their autonomy or undermining their medical au-thority. As the attending on the medical service, I was here to teach, to help, to be ultimately responsible (legally and medically), but also to allow the house staff to learn by making independent decisions.

The challenge was actually enticing, given the hordes of problems that Mr. Karlin offered and the delicate balance the house staff required. I hoped that this would be a chance to teach the subtler aspects of patient care, to demonstrate the skills that an attending can offer, all while completing my own duties in a reasonable time frame. Realizing that I was in for the long haul, I asked if I could sit in the visitors' chair at his bedside.

Mr. Karlin immediately stopped his ranting. "You are the first doctor who's ever sat down," he said in a slower, more thoughtful voice. "Everyone else is always in such a rush."

"I have less on my plate," I replied nonchalantly, pushing away thoughts of the twenty-five patients I had yet to meet. Inside, I was hoping that I'd scored one tiny point for our alliance.

Mr. Karlin proceeded to recatalogue, with further embellishment, the errors, indignities, adversities, and insults that had befallen him since the ambulance had had the temerity to deposit him on the doorstep of this most miserable of all hospitals.

"Mr. Karlin," I said, resisting the impulse to smile, "how about if you tell me the single worst problem that's bothering you right now."

"Oh, you challenge me, Doctor," he said, voice low with concentration. "There are so many possibilities from which to choose." Mr. Karlin paused and wrinkled his brow. "At this precise instant, I'd have to say that the worst problem is my pain. No one is getting me any pain medicines. When the planets align properly and the United Nations Security Council passes a unanimous resolution and I finally *get* a goddamn pain pill, it isn't strong enough and it doesn't last long enough."

Aha! Here's a finite problem that I can solve, I thought to myself. I could order the stronger pain medicines that he needed and get them to him immediately. If I could deliver results that were meaningful to him, I might just be able to get a foothold into a trusting relationship that would allow us, hopefully, to diagnose and treat the cause of his syncope.

I excused myself and consulted Mr. Karlin's tomelike chart. I saw that the medical team had ordered him Tylenol with codeine p.r.n.; that is, he'd get it only when he asked for it.

Residents and interns are notoriously ginger when it comes to pain medications. One advantage to being an attending is that, having worked with these medications for many more years and with many more patients than my residents have, I feel a bit more confident with their use.

I tracked down the intern and suggested that we order morphine injections on a regular standing basis and that we get him the first dose right now. And that we shouldn't even wait for the nurse to pick up the order and then get the medication; we should do it ourselves. The intern watched as I asked the head nurse if she wouldn't mind putting aside what she was doing at that moment to bring me a stat dose of five milligrams of morphine, telling her that it could not wait for the order to be processed via the usual route. Then I marched into Mr. Karlin's room and injected it into his arm, all within ten minutes of his telling me he had pain.

Within fifteen minutes Mr. Karlin was feeling better. Back in the doctors' station, I related my theory of "gaining credibility by using decisive actions" to the house staff. The resident was a bit skeptical. "I think he's just drug-seeking," she said.

"He might be," I answered. "But we have to start from the point of view of believing the patient. If he *says* he has pain, then he *does indeed* have pain, and we should treat that aggressively. If we notice patterns of behavior over the next few days that suggest abusive tendencies, *then* we can reevaluate."

A teaching moment, I thought. A chance to educate the house staff about the importance of treating pain rapidly and forcefully. A satisfying moment in an otherwise hectic first day.

I glanced down my list to see how many more patients were yet to be seen. Still twenty-five more.

By the second day, I was starting to know the ins and outs of the patients, and the ins and outs of the house staff, as we exhaustively and repeatedly reviewed the patient list, debating the pros and cons of each treatment. Mr. Karlin had a lump on his neck that we thought was most likely a bruise from his fall. But we needed to be sure it wasn't an unrelated, and maybe more serious, condition. So far, Mr. Karlin had refused both the CT scan and the MRI because of his claustrophobia, and the resident was getting annoyed. Bellevue didn't possess an open MRI, and there were too many logistical nightmares to transfer him to a hospital that did. Trying to problem-solve for the house staff, I suggested that we do an ultrasound, a procedure that, while a little less accurate, was much easier to tolerate. If Mr. Karlin would agree to that, we'd at least have some information that might help us rule out certain diagnoses.

Several hours later, in the middle of our second review of the day, the intern was paged and informed that Mr. Karlin was refusing the ultrasound of his neck mass. He was down in the radiology suite, but he was apparently putting up a royal fuss.

"He's probably very anxious," I said, thinking decisively, thinking again about solving Mr. Karlin's problem rapidly and definitively, thinking about offering practical solutions to help the house staff. "Grab five milligrams of IV Valium, go down to radiology, and administer it to him before he cancels the test altogether. And bring along some morphine in case he missed his dose of pain meds."

The intern looked at the resident. "You just inject the Valium into the IV?" Her voice was incredulous. The resident nodded.

Another teaching moment. I took the ball: "Of course. It's not a big deal. We give ten milligrams IV for people with seizures and alcohol withdrawal. Five milligrams is a fairly standard dose. Nothing to be afraid of. The main issue is that we shouldn't let him sit there frightened and anxious. We need to address his concerns promptly if we want a chance to gain his trust."

The intern and resident gathered the meds and headed down to radiology.

I then sat down with the other resident to review her patients. We were two-thirds of the way down the list when we heard a code called over the loudspeaker. A reflex of all doctors is to stop in midsentence to hear where the code is taking place. For the resident, it was, of course, crucial. If the code was on one of the medicine floors, she would have to drop everything and run over. For the attending, the reflex was more vestigial, a habit that was impossible to break. Attendings don't participate in codes. Codes are for house staff, who are more nimble and more up to date on the resuscitation protocols.

We both fell silent and cocked our ears. The code announcement was repeated several times, but it was hard to make out what the operator was saying. It sounded like 3-West. Medicine floors are 16 and 17, so we shrugged and went back to our conversation.

It was the clerk who put two and two together. "Three-West, that's ultrasound." He made a quick call. "It's Mr. Karlin who's coding."

Mr. Karlin? My pulse froze.

We dashed to the elevators and waited the agonizing minutes for the stat transport. We made nervous jokes with the anesthesiologist, who was also stuck with us on 16. If the anesthesiologist was with us, that meant he wasn't at the code intubating Mr. Karlin. The minutes ticked on. I could feel a black stone sinking in my stomach.

By the time we got downstairs, there were already crowds of people. I spotted the resident and she called out, "He's fine, don't worry."

Mr. Karlin reached out for my hand, and I clasped it immediately. "What happened?" I asked, trying to hide the panic in my voice.

The resident said, "I injected the Valium, and then he immediately went slack and stopped breathing. We were able to rouse him, but he kept falling back. We injected the antidote to Valium and he woke right back up."

My heart and ego plummeted to the floor. This was clearly my fault. I had, with "decisiveness," told the intern and resident to administer five milligrams of Valium. It was clearly too much for him, despite being a fairly normal dose.

"Have you ever taken Valium before?" I asked Mr. Karlin.

"Sure, tons of times. At least in the pill form."

"Have you ever had a reaction before?"

"No, never," Mr. Karlin said with a wry smile. "But this was a nice chance to say hello to our Creator. Thanks for keeping the greetings brief."

I felt a tad better, knowing he had tolerated Valium before. Maybe it had just been an idiosyncratic reaction. But still, I was the instigator of the events. Causing a code was not a very impressive example for the house staff, certainly not the best way to gain credibility with them. And nearly killing Mr. Karlin was not exactly progress toward forming a doctor-patient alliance.

And this was only day 2 of my month attending on the wards.

For the rest of that week, a low level of anxiety trailed me. We weren't making progress on a diagnosis for Mr. Karlin's syncope, and he was smart enough to know it. His dissatisfaction with every aspect of his hospital course was profound, and he reminded me of it every day. And he was even less interested, now, in pursuing more diagnostic tests. "You already killed me once, thank you very much," he'd say. "I'll pass on this next opportunity." I could detect hints of an affable charm seeping through his crotchety veneer, but it didn't make our encounters any easier.

I began to feel an urgency about Mr. Karlin. I felt that he was slipping from us—not in an acute medical way, but in a serious manner nonetheless. We were rapidly losing his faith both in us and in the system.

The odd thing was that I didn't sense the same urgency from the house staff. They were certainly eager to find the correct diagnosis, both from a medical standpoint and also to move Mr. Karlin along toward discharge, to keep their patient rosters from burgeoning. This was something that Mr. Karlin clearly intuited and was not afraid to articulate on a regular basis.

"You folks just want to get me discharged," he said on morning rounds, running his hand though his gray-white hair, greasy from three weeks of hospital stay.

"Well, we've done every test that we can think of," the resident said. "Sometimes the cause of syncope is never found. But at least we've ruled out all the serious causes."

A less perceptive or more timid patient might have found that answer somewhat reassuring. Not Mr. Karlin.

"You think you can just push me along, check me off on your list, and get on with your other work. First you try to kill me, then you try to kick me out. I'm a lot smarter than your average patient. I know there's a Patients' Bill of Rights somewhere in my nightstand, but I can't read it because my bed light doesn't work. But that doesn't matter because I still haven't gotten my glaucoma drops. And none of that matters a piff in this world because my reading glasses are gone. Just 1.5 lousy diopters! That's all I ask for in this life, but you guys just want to give me the boot."

Mr. Karlin was both annoying and pitiable in his rage. I sympathized with him, but it was also growing increasingly difficult to spend time in his room. With nearly forty patients to visit every day, even five minutes per patient meant that rounds lasted three hours. Mr. Karlin routinely kept me in his room for nearly half an hour. When we talked about things other than the hospital and the abysmal care he was receiving, Mr. Karlin's sarcasm would lift, ever so briefly. I wished that I didn't have so many duties pulling me elsewhere so we could just sit and chat. But inevitably, the conversation would drift back to his seemingly unsolvable medical situation. I would feel my body begin to twitch with frustration, my fingers start to jitter, my legs grow restless, until the sensation would bubble over, and I'd have to escape the room.

Mr. Karlin was sensitive about being ignored, and I realized how important it was for me not to appear rushed with him. I certainly *wanted* to take my time with him, and our nonmedical conversations could be interesting, but there was no way to avoid the sensation of all my day's work pressing down on my shoulders. Nonetheless, I made myself sit down in the chair each day with him, determined to offer him this bit of respect, determined not to slip into the inevitable body language that suggests that one might rather be elsewhere. It wasn't that Mr. Karlin was an unpleasant person—there was an amiable grouchiness about him—but day in and day out it was exhausting to listen to him rant about things that I seemed powerless to solve. His tirades constantly reminded me of our limitations, our inabilities, our errors, the inhumanity of the system.

And rant he did. At times I couldn't tell what was true and what was fantasy. He talked about being a lecturer who traveled around the world speaking at all the major universities, of having attended several major universities, of completing a doctorate, of attending law school. He spoke of having his writings and his art published. He spoke of being an entrepreneur, of founding several technology companies.

This seemed hard to reconcile with the scrawny man who possessed a world-weariness not too different from that of our homeless patients. There was that slight wild look in his face, the hollow cheeks, chaotic eyebrows, angular bones. I knew from the ambulance report that his apartment was so cluttered with junk that it had been nearly impossible for the paramedics to get to him. He didn't seem to have any human connections; no friends, coworkers, or family that I ever saw, though he did mention a daughter who lived far away.

He spoke repeatedly about a doctor he had been seeing, "a world-famous expert on nerves," who was giving him monthly intravenous infusions of protein for his nerves. The house staff rolled their eyes when he talked about this, and I, too, was a bit skeptical. Monthly IV infusions of protein sounded like something a less-than-scrupulous alternative healer might do. It certainly didn't make any clinical sense to me.

"He's an expert; all the other doctors come to him for advice," Mr. Karlin insisted.

Mr. Karlin could give me a name, but no phone number, for this doctor. There was no phone number when I called the operator, adding to my suspicions that this was all rather farfetched. An Internet search, however, revealed an e-mail address for that doctor. Maybe there was some truth to his story. I sent an e-mail but never received a reply.

I tried to explain to the house staff why the potential loss of Mr. Karlin's trust was so critical, but it seemed that this was something I could only feel, not explain. I knew that I had to approach Mr. Karlin on two levels: I had to find a way to make a personal connection, and I had to help make a satisfying medical diagnosis. But I also knew that there was a very good chance that we would *not* be able to make a diagnosis (as happens so often with syncope), and that I'd have to build a reserve of trust with him in order to convince him of this.

A snowstorm was raging one day during Mr. Karlin's third week on 16-West. New York City doesn't usually get major snowstorms until January or February, if at all, but here it was, a full-fledged blizzard even before the winter solstice. It was wet, slushy, and windy. Even my more intrepid colleagues, the ones who managed to go out for lunch every single day, were settling in for the daily special at the Bellevue coffee shop. But I needed to run over to the VA hospital for a meeting.

Just before I scooted out the door that day, with my down jacket, scarf, hat, and gloves, I checked on a new patient who'd been admitted that morning for chest pain. Mr. Medina was a slight man in his sixties, whose Dominican Spanish I found nearly unintelligible. But he had a winning smile, and when I entered his room I saw that he had been doodling on paper towels. Three brown paper towels were laid out on his bedside table, and a progression of flowers and vines and animals was exploding on the rough surfaces. I dug in my pockets, looking for better paper to give him. All I had were a few sheets of pink progress notes, but he was grateful for something more substantial than paper towels.

In awkward Spanish, I elicited his medical history of chest pain. I also learned that he was an amateur watercolorist. I made sure that his medications were in order, and then I dashed out of Bellevue into the whirling snowstorm.

I slid through the icy paths of the Bellevue garden, past the fountain and the sundial. The traffic of First Avenue was audibly and visually muted by the storm, and the stately wrought-iron fence that surrounded the garden seemed to block out the modern world. For one brief moment I felt transported back to nineteenth-century New York, but then an ambulance siren blared into my reverie and I was reminded of the drab twenty-first-century meeting that was the reason for this outing.

I slogged my way through the slush toward the VA hospital. Across the street I noticed a pharmacy. I was, as usual, running late, but was still struck by the image of Mr. Medina's artistic talents being squandered on paper towels and pink progress notes. So I decided to take a slight detour, decided that it was important enough to spare a few minutes. The pounding icy snow bit into my face as I crossed the street. I wished I'd brought an umbrella but realized that it would have been useless. I ducked inside the pharmacy and searched the aisles till I found the stationery supplies. There was a small children's watercolor set. I grabbed it, along with a pad of drawing paper and some extra brushes. As I went to pay for these, I saw a display of reading glasses.

Suddenly I remembered Mr. Karlin's conversation from our first day, about how his reading glasses had been lost in the ambulance. I know that I can't stand even waiting for an elevator without something to read; I couldn't imagine what it would feel like to be stuck in a hospital bed for weeks, unable to read. Just 1.5 lousy diopters, he'd said. I reached for a pair of reading glasses—choosing the black wire-rimmed over the faux tortoiseshell—and then continued my interhospital hike in the whipping wet snow.

Mr. Medina was delighted with the paints (and two weeks after his discharge, a framed painting arrived in my clinic). Mr. Karlin, when I gave him the reading glasses, broke out in the first grudging smile I'd seen since we met. Along with his glasses, I offered him the most recent issue of the *Bellevue Literary Review,* so he'd have something to read other than the Patients' Bill of Rights. He seemed genuinely impressed that our hospital housed a literary magazine. "Maybe you aren't all heathens after all," he said. "Aside from the fact that you nearly killed me, and that you can't figure out my diagnosis, and that you won't give me my protein infusions, maybe you aren't such barbarians after all."

Mr. Karlin warmed up to us much more after that. He wasn't quite as cranky on rounds and seemed more willing to listen to what the house staff had to say. But while we'd made some progress on a human connection with him, we still hadn't figured out the cause of his syncope.

Reading through thick charts of patients who've already been in the hospital for some time is an arduous task. It is obviously important, but it takes inordinate patience (and time) to sift though pages and pages of scrawled notes and to piece together the data, some of which are in the computer, some of which are in one section of the chart, some of which are buried in another section, and some of which exist only in the heads of the doctors who don't take time to write detailed—or legible—notes.

While paging through Mr. Karlin's chart, I could see that he'd had most of the usual tests for syncope: a sonogram of the heart, a twenty-four-hour EKG monitor, an ultrasound of his carotid arteries, a CT scan of his brain. He'd refused the cardiac stress test because the machine that would take pictures of his chest made him claustrophobic (and I had no intention of giving him any more Valium for anxiety!). The mass on his neck turned out, as we'd thought, to be a hematoma, a collection of blood that was probably a result of having fallen on the floor in his home. It had begun to recede, and he was asking for slightly less pain medication.

I realized that we'd never checked an EEG (electroencephalogram) to evaluate him for seizures, which can be a cause of syncope, though it usually presents with the classic full-body shaking of a grand mal seizure. I also realized that it might be time to officially consult neurology, since Mr. Karlin reported *repeated* episodes of syncope, not just one isolated occurrence.

Meanwhile, the hospital case managers were pressuring us to begin planning Mr. Karlin's discharge. His insurance would soon stop paying for his hospitalization. Mr. Karlin was quite weak from his hospital stay, and it seemed as though he'd been frail even before he was admitted to the hospital. At this point, he couldn't even walk. It was clear that Mr. Karlin would need to go to a rehabilitation facility for a few weeks before he could return home, if he even *could* return home. In his current state, he looked like a candidate for a nursing home.

The physical therapists came to work with Mr. Karlin daily, but these were not always successful encounters. The therapist would tell me that Mr. Karlin was rather stubborn and that if he couldn't accomplish one exercise, he'd give up immediately. Mr. Karlin told me that the therapists always managed to come at the wrong time, with the wrong attitude, and refused to be flexible in rescheduling.

When I tried to speak to Mr. Karlin about the possibility of going to a rehabilitation facility upon discharge—I wanted to give him as much advance warning as possible—he immediately got his hackles up. "You guys just want to throw me out and get on with your lives. Once I'm shipped off to this rehab place, you'll cross my name off your list and not expend another brain cell in my direction."

I couldn't help but feel ashamed, because I knew there were aspects of truth to his words: once patients left the hospital, we did not, indeed, think much about them. This wasn't because we didn't care about them, or hadn't cared about them, but more a consequence of the fact that thirty new patients would arrive and occupy our emotional and logistical energy. The intense and rapid-fire connections were almost like serial one-night stands, except there were thirty one-night stands happening simultaneously, followed by thirty new ones, on an ongoing, exhausting basis. This reality could not be avoided. But it did sound callous when it was articulated in plain English.

"And how can you even think of discharging me before you know what's wrong with me?" Mr. Karlin demanded in his characteristic style that incited both sympathy and defensiveness.

I explained, once again, that medical science was imperfect, and that sometimes there were conditions—syncope was one of them —for which we could not find an ironclad diagnosis. But that we were ruling out the serious cardiovascular and neurological causes.

I felt like I was parroting a party line. Even though it was all technically true, it ran rough in my mouth. There was something so impersonal, so dismissive in it. But I didn't have anything better to offer.

"Knowing what you *don't* have is not particularly reassuring," Mr. Karlin said. "And no one's giving me my IV protein. Besides, I'm not ready for rehab yet. I can't even walk."

Ignoring the fact that we could not locate an address or phone number for his "world-famous" doctor, I gently explained that not being able to walk was the very reason he would be going to rehab. I also gingerly mentioned that once the medical evaluation was finished, his insurance company would be unlikely to cover his hospitalization.

"Aha, so that's it. It's all about money." He rolled his sunken eyes up to the ceiling. "This place is pitiful."

"Mr. Karlin," I said. "I hate, more than anything, having to talk about money, but if your insurance company doesn't cover your stay, then you will be faced with a monstrous bill when you get home. If I didn't warn you about the realities of the system, I'd be remiss in my duties.

"It unfortunately doesn't matter whether I agree with it or not, it's just one of those rules that we have to live by. And even though we don't have a diagnosis yet, and possibly may never find a diagnosis, we still have to plan for what happens after you leave the hospital."

"Don't I get a chance to get used to the idea?" he said, still talking to the ceiling. "I mean, are you just going to toss me out?"

"The way the process works," I explained, "is that the social worker will locate several rehab facilities that will accept your insurance. Then you or a family member can visit them and decide which one you want..."

Mr. Karlin cocked his face toward me. The raggedness of his face seemed even more exaggerated than when we'd first met. "Do I *look* like I'm in any condition to go visiting rehabs?"

I squirmed in my chair. "Well, that's the theory, anyway. You get to pick a few and we'll apply to them. Then, the first one that has a bed available—"

"—You ship me out before the lunch trays come."

"Well, not quite, but once your insurance company knows that there is a rehab spot available to you, they will stop paying your hospital bills."

"Money, money. You guys are all about money." With obvious effort, he twisted his body away from me to stare at the curtain separating him from his roommate, who was moaning from painful pancreatitis.

The last thing I wanted to do was be the mouthpiece for a Byzantine, illogical, often unfair health-care system, but here I was passing along the corporate policy, and I had to admit, it sounded pretty utilitarian. "I'm sorry," I said. "I really am. I wish the system weren't like this."

There was a pause, and the whir of the radiator and the buzz of the overhead lights suddenly seemed to swarm the room and invade my ears. Then Mr. Karlin whipped his head back toward me with more force than I'd seen him generate since I'd known him in the hospital. "Don't you get it?" he said. "Don't you get it?" he asked again. "I'm scared! As awful as this cesspool of a hospital is, at least I know what I'm up against. Who knows what awaits me in some crummy rehab? At least the crumminess here is familiar, even a bit homey." Tears began to well up in the crusted corners of his eyes, and his voice grew more gruff.

I reached out for his hand, which was half hidden by the muss of his bed sheets. His skin was dry and parchment-thin. It didn't seem strong enough to protect him from the justifiable and real fears that he faced.

"I know what's going to happen," he continued in a hacking voice. "They'll find some rehab place in East Nowheresville, and then haul my corpus onto a stretcher and wheel me off. And I'm too damn weak to fight you all off."

That haunting image hung in my head for the rest of the day. What would it feel like to have one's body transported to a new location, against one's will, and not have the physical power to protest?

The next day I went to Mr. Karlin's room and found a young neurology resident finishing her evaluation. On Mr. Karlin's nightstand were his reading glasses, his now well-worn copy of the *Bellevue Literary Review*, and, to my surprise, a copy of my first book, *Singular Intimacies: Becoming a Doctor at Bellevue*.

As a rule, I try to be conscientious about separating my clinical life from my literary life, and I rarely discuss my writing when I am working with patients. But there it was, my book—my *baby*—sitting on Mr. Karlin's nightstand.

"Hey," I said, feeling a goofy grin slide across my face, "how did you get that?"

"Well," Mr. Karlin said with a bit of obvious self-satisfaction, "Dr. Handler revealed your secret and then kindly offered to loan me her copy."

Dr. Handler, the neurology resident, was a petite, sweet-faced woman with sleek black hair pulled back into a ponytail. We introduced ourselves and shook hands.

"And she's also given me the most thorough exam I've had since I've been here," Mr. Karlin added. "The food still sucks in this place, and the nurses still don't answer my calls, but my opinion of the medical staff here has gone up by a few notches, though it's still way in the negative-number zone."

"And you are very lucky," said Dr. Handler, "because Dr. Brodsky, the chairman of neurology, is on service this month, so he'll be coming to see you this afternoon."

When I saw Mr. Karlin later on that day, he was positively beaming. His reading glasses were pushed up on top of his head, and he had three books, plus the newspaper, sprawled out on his bed. "Dr. Brodsky," he said, with palpable awe in his voice, "now *that's* a doctor!"

"I guess they didn't make him chairman for nothing," I replied.

"You should have seen him." Mr. Karlin sounded like he was relating the tie-breaking play in the World Series. "He came in here with a whole posse of doctors, so many that they could barely fit. He spent nearly an hour here, was even more thorough than Dr. Handler. And he was a true gentleman. And you know what else? He's the first guy around here that I've seen wearing a tie—a bow tie, no less. Your crew of doctors is a pretty rangy bunch."

I stopped and thought about that for a moment, then realized that Mr. Karlin was right; the house staff did look rather scruffy. Maybe it was already becoming a generational thing, but when I was a resident, on non-call days the men wore shirts and ties. Now as I gazed at the residents and interns on my ward, I realized that they dressed every day as though they were on call, wearing scrubs and sneakers. I realized that I had not seen a single one of the men wear a tie all month. The women were dressed casually as well.

"I used to give lectures on professionalism," Mr. Karlin said, "and I think your motley crew could use a lesson or two."

Within two days, Dr. Brodsky proposed a working diagnosis for Mr. Karlin. "Pan-dysautonomia," Dr. Handler reported to us. "It's an autoimmune disorder that affects the peripheral nerves. There's an inherited version that kids get, but occasionally it can be seen in adults. We'll have to send some blood samples to the Mayo Clinic in Rochester for verification—they have a specialized research lab—but Dr. Brodsky feels quite sure about this."

The treatment, it turned out, was intravenous infusions of gamma globulin—a mixture of the body's antibody proteins.

"You guys are brilliant," Mr. Karlin said, waving a skeletal arm in the air. "Three weeks, a million tests, a gajillion dollars, a special chance to nearly meet my Maker, only to give me the same goddamn treatment I've been getting every month from my own specialist."

He was right. It seemed that his famed doctor had indeed diagnosed him with an autoimmune neurological disorder and had been giving him the appropriate treatment—the intravenous protein Mr. Karlin had been talking about. We just hadn't listened to him or taken him seriously. And Dr. Handler told us that Dr. Brodsky, the chairman, immediately recognized the name of the specialist, who was indeed renowned in his field.

Though we doctors routinely disparage the paternalism of days past, it was clear that we still unconsciously engaged in a good deal of it. It was almost impossible for our team of educated doctors to give credence to the opinions of this wisp of a man who didn't look like he knew what he was talking about.

And though we now have Internet access all over the hospital, and though I'd even used it to try to find Mr. Karlin's specialist, it had never dawned on me to do an Internet search on Mr. Karlin himself. Somehow my brain couldn't process those two concepts—Mr. Karlin and the Internet—within the same synapse.

I finished my time on the ward just before Mr. Karlin went to rehab, and I spent a long time saying good-bye. Dr. Handler had given him her copy of my book, and I was honored when he asked me to autograph it.

A week later I sat down to write this essay. And it wasn't until I was near the end—until I wrote the above paragraph, in fact—that it finally dawned on me that I should try an Internet search on Mr. Karlin.

I typed in "Lester Karlin" and he popped right up on the computer screen. Everything he'd said was true, or at least partially true. He was an entrepreneur, had started two companies, had developed technology for a particular aspect of electronic commerce. He had attended several Ivy League universities, though his Ph.D. was honorary. He had attended law school but didn't actually complete a degree. His articles were cited, and he had even been inducted into a hall of fame in the electronic business world.

Most of these citations were from more than a decade ago, and there were no recent mentions. I finally met his daughter when she flew in to help arrange his affairs. It seemed that Mr. Karlin had been very successful in the business world for a time, but then things had unraveled. Even she couldn't say why, having moved with her mother, at age four, to the Midwest. Occasional visits over the years had given her glimpses of her father's life but never a full picture.

Is it institutional blindness, I've often wondered, that makes it so difficult for doctors to envision patients beyond their role as sick people? When we gaze at our patients in those awful blue gowns, camped on that ultimate symbol of infirmity, the hospital bed, it seems impossible that they ever had other lives. We can't imagine them running for the subway, balancing a checkbook, shouting down an underling, changing light bulbs, having sex. Is our vision clouded because we are so immersed in the world of sickness? Is it because this helps reinforce the power dynamic that has kept patients "in their place" for centuries? Or might it be because, like Mr. Karlin, we doctors are scared down to our bones? If we were to see our patients living the lives that we live, then there would be nothing to separate them from us. And then we could easily become them.

And so we squint, keeping our focus on that narrow sliver of sickness. Until someone like Mr. Karlin retrieves our glasses for us.

CHAPTER EIGHT

Terminal Thoughts

"Ms. Binet is refusing dialysis." Kimberly sighed. "We can't get anything done with her." Kimberly was the second-year resident—the PGY-II, or postgraduate year two—running the medical service with her team of interns. After a few months in the clinic, I was back on the wards once again as the attending on 16-North. Ms. Binet had been intermittently refusing various procedures—blood draws, IVs, X-rays—but for dialysis this was a first. Without it, the body's toxins would accumulate, and death would occur in a matter of days.

"She doesn't want dialysis?" I asked.

"No," Kimberly said. "She said she's had enough."

I nodded slowly. One of the tricky parts of being a supervising attending was allowing the residents enough autonomy to learn how to make decisions while still ensuring proper medical care. It was always hard for me to resist the impulse to simply do what I thought was best. "What do you think we should do?"

"Her brother and his wife will be visiting during lunch, and I thought we'd have a family meeting to discuss it." Kimberly gathered her sleek black hair into a ponytail.

Ms. Binet was a frail seventy-nine-year-old woman; she was originally from Salonika but she had lived in America for more than thirty years. When I came on service this week she had been battling both pancreatitis and peritonitis. Because of her inflamed pancreas, she hadn't been allowed to eat for almost two weeks, and her 110-pound body had withered to 85 pounds. Intravenous nutrition was tried, but she suffered the side effects of infection and fluid overload. And fluid overload was the last thing she needed, since her kidneys were damaged and could not urinate out the excess. Dialysis was a daily ordeal to remove enough of the fluid so that she could breathe comfortably but not so much that she'd drop her blood pressure, which had already happened several times. Ms. Binet broke out in a full-body rash from one antibiotic, and got severe itching from another. Everything we did seemed to cause another problem.

I breathed a sigh of relief. "Excellent idea, Kimberly. Ms. Binet has been through a lot and I think it would be best to discuss such heavy decisions with her family present. Do you feel comfortable handling this discussion yourself, or would you like me to participate?"

Kimberly thought for a moment. "I think I can do it myself, Dr. Ofri," she said, tucking her index cards into her pocket. She was, after all, a second-year resident, halfway through her training.

"I have confidence in you," I said, not entirely sure if I believed myself. But how can someone learn if not by actually doing? "I'm sure you can handle it, but feel free to page me if you need some help." Always a balance with the residents.

━━━⁌⁌⁍⁍━━━

Kimberly returned a few hours later. "We had a discussion, the four of us. Ms. Binet was clear that she doesn't want to do any more dialysis, even if it means she will die. She is very definite about her wishes. We signed a DNR and will now work toward hospice."

"Good job," I said instinctively. I was always relieved when a patient came to their own terms about the limits of medical treatment and we could focus on making them comfortable instead of torturing them with unending procedures. "I'll cosign the DNR as soon as I'm finished here."

I went back to the chart I was working on, completing my comments on Mr. Preston's pneumonia. Kimberly was checking the day's lab results in the computer. After five minutes I looked up and stared into the empty X-ray light box. The grayish-white plastic was scratched and mottled from at least two decades' worth of films being rammed into the clips. They were the same light boxes that were in the doctors' stations when I had been a medical student, intern, and then resident. When I did my first medical-student rotation—in this very doctors' station on 16-North, as a matter of fact—the light boxes were already worn out.

There is an inimitable slapping sound when an X-ray is slid onto the light box, a crack when it inserts itself into the clips on top. Then the fluorescent whir as the background light trundles awake, triggered by the X-ray, flickering languidly before finally illuminating the film. Those sounds and sensations were becoming extinct; computerized X-rays had begun to take over. While access to X-rays at any computer has distinct advantages over endless hunting for lost films (usually confiscated by the surgeons!), there is a generation of doctors-in-training who will never know the silky feeling of sliding an X-ray onto a light box and the satisfying click as it locks into place. Now the light box serves mainly as a place to post notes, lab results, and Chinese take-out menus.

"Hospice," I said slowly, not to anyone in particular, as I gazed at the light box. I kneaded the word over my tongue as my eyes drifted around the doctors' station, with its chaotic piles of charts and lab slips and used coffee cups. Hospice—one of the revolutions in medicine in the past twenty years, the humane way to ease suffering. Hospice—I craned my neck upward, running through my list of patients in my head. I'd been learning thirty-four patients—half of whom were Kimberly's—over the past few days. I'd been reading their charts, but the truth was I didn't have every detail down yet, especially the ones like Ms. Binet with hospital courses that were tortuous and complicated. "Hospice," I said again. I recalled that breast cancer was in Ms. Binet's history. "What is the state of Ms. Binet's breast cancer?" I wondered aloud.

"Uh, I'm not sure," Kimberly said, looking up from the computer. "It hasn't come up in this hospital stay." She went back to copying down the results.

"Is it metastatic? Or recurrent?"

"Umm, I'm not sure," she said, this time not looking up. "I could check if you want," she added with enough passivity in her voice to make it clear that she really wished I'd leave her alone.

Hospice—the concept that I so embraced and promoted. Why was it sticking on my tongue? "Kimberly," I said, interrupting her work yet again, "what exactly *is* Ms. Binet's terminal illness?"

"Well, she's pretty end-stage," Kimberly said almost defensively, with a knowing tone in her voice— a tone that not just invited but almost compelled me to agree with the obvious. And I couldn't disagree with her entirely—Ms. Binet looked as cachectic and near-death as any of our cancer patients.

I didn't answer, still envisioning Ms. Binet: frail body, assiduously dyed blond hair, proper European bearings despite all manner of bodily insults. Horribly ill. But terminal?

Kimberly picked up on my hesitation, my evident dissatisfaction with her answer. "She's got end-stage renal disease," she offered in a less defensive tone, hoping, I sensed, that this would satisfy me and thus bring an end to this conversation and to my annoying questions.

"I know, but dialysis for end-stage renal disease is different than other life-sustaining treatments. People can live for *decades* with dialysis." I could see Kimberly's expression stiffening, and I decided to back off a bit. We had to work together and to rely on each other for a whole month. I didn't want to start out in a contentious manner. "Kimberly, I commend you for identifying pain as one of Ms. Binet's most important issues, and you're right that we should be much more aggressive with pain control. But I do need to know: What is Ms. Binet's *terminal* illness for which she should be in a hospice?"

Kimberly was silent.

I left Kimberly and walked over to the nurses' station. From the chart rack I hauled out Ms. Binet's voluminous chart, which I had skimmed earlier in the week. Like Mr. Karlin's, it was the type of chart that one approaches with dread: spilling over with progress notes, consult sheets, X-ray reports, nursing notes. Weeks of handling by so many people had torn the ring-holes in many of the sheets, leaving them poking out awkwardly, their edges bending and tearing from the abuse. I started at the beginning and slowly, agonizingly, sifted through the endless notes, penned in the chicken scrawl that typifies most interns.

Ms. Binet had a complicated medical history. Her osteoporosis left her with multiple fractures and chronic pain. There was hypertension and diabetes, both of which damaged the kidneys. She had coronary disease with an old heart attack and a tendency to accumulate fluid in her lungs. Her dialysis had been complicated by multiple episodes of abdominal infections. There was breast cancer treated several years ago but no mention—at least that I could find—of recurrence or spread. And there was the current bout of pancreatitis that was making her miserable, with crampy abdominal pain and strict orders from the surgeons not to eat in order that her bowel could rest. All chronic conditions. All horrible. But *terminal?* She reminded me of Mr. Reston, in that small Florida town, but without the overarching depression that had made him suicidal.

Ms. Binet was a fragile-appearing woman with cropped blond hair and gold wire-rimmed glasses bearing her initials, MB, at the edge of one lens. Her thin body seemed nearly melted into the bed as I looked in from the doorway of her room. Next to her sat her brother, a squat, balding man with a round face and a worn sports jacket. His wife immediately gave up her chair to me when I entered, over my protests.

I introduced myself to the family then faced Ms. Binet. "Dr. Lee tells me that you've had enough with dialysis."

Ms. Binet scrunched her dry lips and stared at me for a moment before speaking. "I've had enough, period." Her voice was quiet, with a faint European accent that rounded and parsed her words. "Every time I blink there's another person with a needle to take my blood, another X-ray, another this, another that. And always dialysis. Dialysis, dialysis, and more dialysis." She closed her eyes for a moment. Even just those sentences seemed to tire her.

"Do you understand what would happen if you stopped dialysis?" I asked.

"It would be 'So long, Charlie' for me," she said with a rueful smile.

I couldn't help a small chuckle from coming through. There was a certain charm about her, about her ability to choose such an American expression, one that was almost frivolous, in the face of such a grim topic. It was as though illness could debilitate her body but not her ironic wit. "You're right," I answered. "Without kidneys or dialysis you would die within a week."

"See, Marianne," the brother broke in, pressing forward in his chair. "You can't do this. You will die. Tell her, Doctor. Make her understand."

"Ms. Binet," I said, "I'm not here to talk you out of your decision. As far as I'm concerned, if you've decided to stop dialysis, that is your wish and I will respect it." The brother flopped back against his seat. "I just would like to understand what you are feeling, if that's okay." She nodded. "Stopping dialysis means you are going to die. Do you want to die?"

"I don't want to live anymore, if that's what you're asking."

I let those words settle. Then I decided to engage her on this, not mock her or point out the intrinsic illogic, but take her words at their value. I was genuinely curious how she felt about this and also acutely aware that her life was truly at stake. "Let's say I had a gun right here," I said, as matter-of-factly as I could. "Would you shoot yourself?" I could sense both the brother and sister-in-law stiffen.

"Too messy. I'm not the messy type."

"How about a bottle of pills?" I pressed. "Would you take them and just get it all over with?"

"No, guns and pills are all too fast. I want to die slowly." Ms. Binet sighed. "A week is a good time."

The sister-in-law stepped forward and punctuated the air with her hands as she spoke. "See, Doctor, she doesn't know what she's talking about. She can't stop dialysis just because she *feels* like it."

Ignoring her, I continued to focus on Ms. Binet. "Do you have any hope for the future?" I asked, probing for clinical signs of depression.

"What is there to hope for?" Ms. Binet replied dryly. "Except to die sooner."

I didn't seem to be getting very far; Marianne Binet had a well-constructed reply for everything. I suspected that Ms. Binet might be suffering from depression, but depression is often hard to distinguish from realistic pessimism. Standard signs of depression such as loss of appetite and poor sleep appear in many chronically ill patients who are not depressed.

I tried the most straightforward approach to diagnosis. "Do *you* think you are depressed?"

"Of course I am," she said, fixing her eyes on me. "Wouldn't you be?"

I didn't have an answer for that one and suddenly felt self-conscious about my own good health. I could feel an urgency gathering at the back of my throat and I had to take two slow breaths to calm my voice.

"Tell me, Ms. Binet," I said, trying again. "What is the worst part about being here in the hospital?"

"Which worst do you want?" she said. "The pain? The fact that I can't eat? The fact that I am on antibiotics around the clock? The fact that I get stuck with needles every day? The fact that dialysis makes me miserable? The fact that I am here at all? They're all the worst."

Again I was silenced. The sheer enormity and variety of the ways in which illness and medicine inflicted misery on patients was astounding. Mr. Karlin certainly pressed that point home with me. Anything I could say would be puny in comparison.

But I had to say something. I couldn't let nihilism win the day, even if it did seem pretty damn logical at the moment.

"What if we could take care of your pain?" I tried, knowing that this was a promise I wasn't sure we could fulfill.

"You can't," she said, her voice a shade more defiant now. "The little pain medicines don't work and the big ones make me so constipated that it's just as bad as the pain." Her fingers crept toward her belly almost instinctively.

"What if we could give you something for the constipation?"

"Those red pills don't work and the liquid is disgusting. And don't give me any enemas. This place is awful and my loving family here wants to toss me into the nearest nursing home. And my insurance barely covers any of this."

I clearly wasn't getting anywhere. Like Mr. Karlin, Ms. Binet was sharp as a razor. She saw that so many of our treatments were weak nostrums that often made things worse rather than better. She knew that we in the medical profession were miserably inadequate at dealing with complex chronic illnesses that intersected with social woes and economic constraints. And she was freely willing to give up on us, and give up on herself.

I leaned back in my chair. "So it looks like we haven't done such a good job so far." Ms. Binet nodded, triumphant to have scored a point. "But we do have pain experts in the hospital," I added. "I'd like them to come see you, if that's okay, whether or not you continue dialysis. They often come up with much better combinations of things for pain and constipation."

Ms. Binet shrugged. "But I'm still stuck in this damned hospital." Her voice rose now. "And I don't want a nursing home. I'd rather be hung."

"She can't take care of herself," the sister-in-law said. "Look how weak she is. And we live too far away. We can't be there every day."

"See?" Ms. Binet waved her hand in the air. "They want to dump me in a home."

"What if," I said, "we could get the right amount of nursing care for you to be in your own home?"

"The social worker says my insurance only covers four hours a day."

I was sinking into a quagmire. This was impossible, but I had no choice but to keep at it. If I quit, Ms. Binet would be dead by the weekend.

"Hmm...sometimes reality is pretty awful," I said, nodding my head slowly. "I just wonder sometimes..." Ms. Binet looked slantwise at me. "Let's just pretend for a second. Let's say we could figure out the right medicines to take away your pain."

"Can't be done." Ms. Binet cut me off.

"Okay, but humor me for a moment. Let's just say we had some magic pills that would work. You wouldn't have pain and there'd be no constipation." Ms. Binet eyed me warily. "And let's say we worked out a way for you to go home. Let's say the insurance company would cover enough home nursing such that you would be comfortable." Still no reply. "And you could eat regular food again."

Ms. Binet contemplated the ceiling.

"*If* we could do all those things," I said, "and I know that's a big if—but if we could, do you think you might want to live?"

"But you can't do all those things," Ms. Binet insisted, and I knew she was probably right.

"Play along with me for just a moment," I persisted, knowing that I didn't have anything else to offer. "Let's pretend we could. Would you be interested in living some more if you were at home, eating your own food, without any pain?"

Ms. Binet shrugged faintly. "I suppose. Maybe."

There it was—the creak of the castle door that I'd been longing for. The faintest glimpse of a view into Ms. Binet's heart. I could feel the breath warm in my throat as my muscles untensed. "I admit that we haven't done such a good job so far, especially in the pain department." I looked into her eyes and I could see the azure irises that were hiding behind her thick glasses. "Would you be willing to give us a second chance? A chance to do it better."

Ms. Binet shrugged again. "Maybe."

"The pain experts could come by tomorrow. The medicines they recommend, though, could take a few days to work. Usually we spend a week or so adjusting the doses until we find the right combination for each individual patient." I eyed her carefully, but there was no indication of refusal. "At the same time, I'd like to talk with the social worker. Sometimes there are arrangements that we aren't aware of, even the insurance companies aren't aware of. But it often takes a few days or weeks to work out the kinks." Still no rejection. "I can't promise that we can make it all happen instantly—or at all—but I can promise that we will give it a college try."

Ms. Binet nodded ever so slightly, and I took a deep breath. "But we do need a little bit of time," I said. "Would you be willing to continue dialysis at least for a week while we get cracking at this?"

"Will I be able to eat?"

Pancreatitis and the surgeon's orders forbidding food versus negotiating against imminent death and earning credibility with the patient. All of these arrows zinged in my head but I had to make a decision and it would have to be the right one. As the attending on the service, my decision would trump all others—a thought that both inspired and terrified me. "Yes," I said finally. "You may certainly eat."

"Okay, Miss Doctor. Dialysis for a week. I guess I can do that." Ms. Binet pursed her lips lightly. "But I still want my DNR."

"Absolutely. If you know that you never want a breathing tube or shocks on your chest we'll honor that decision. But that doesn't have any effect on dialysis or working on your pain and your home care."

"And my food?"

"*And* your food. If there's not a meal tray here by six, dinner's on me."

———

I made my way down the long and cavernous hall back to the doctors' station. The cheerful designs on the walls combined with the patterned linoleum from the latest renovation gave me a touch of vertigo. I always felt slightly uneasy after I'd convinced a patient to change his or her mind. Despite the professed ideal that we walk into a room with a blank slate, it's never that way. I always have my opinion about what I think should be done, whether it is about DNR, chemotherapy, refusing treatment, withdrawing life-sustaining measures. It's an additional tool, hidden in the pocket of my white coat.

This power makes me feel guilty. We are not really equal at the table.

My discussion with Ms. Binet was the opposite of what usually occurs with such frail patients. Usually I am talking them *out* of medical procedures, helping them see the futility of resuscitation or treatment, not talking them *into* something. This added to my sense of imbalance.

When I arrived at the doctors' station I explained to Kimberly that Ms. Binet would continue dialysis for now while we worked on her pain management and home care issues.

Kimberly shrugged. "Sounds good to me," she said. She made a quick notation on one of her index cards then went back to her work at the computer.

I stood there, waiting for her to say something more, to agree or disagree with my change in her plans. But Kimberly was studiously copying down lab values, one hand on the mouse, the other jotting the numbers on her cards.

I was stunned by her calmness, as though either outcome would have been reasonable. Didn't she see that we'd just had a near-miss experience, or rather a near-death experience? That the options of stopping versus continuing dialysis portended such vastly different outcomes?

And what if I hadn't been here? What if we were still in the old system, the one under which I had trained, in which the residents ran the show entirely? Attendings served more like consultants, showing up for only two hours a day to hear about the new admissions but never following the patients afterward. In that system Ms. Binet would have been dead in a few days.

I recognized, and even applauded, Kimberly's attempts to respect patient autonomy and decision-making, but she simply had not been able to sift through the subtle complexities of depression and frustration in a *chronically* ill patient and understand how that is different than the *terminally* ill patient.

But was it more than that? I was profoundly shaken by the entire episode, but Kimberly seemed to see it as an either/or situation. Maybe she was too bogged down in the myriad details that cloud a resident's life in the hospital, and a patient's refusal of treatment was just one less task to worry about. Did her concern with the logistics of care overshadow her sense of compassion, or did she simply not care one way or the other?

Compassion certainly isn't a requirement to get admitted to medical school, but one hopes that at least a grain already exists and can be developed over time. I often wonder if our method of training doctors serves to stamp out—or at least strain—their innate compassion. When you have a thousand tasks on your scut list to accomplish, one patient's vacillations can throw a wrench into the system. If one patient needs an hour of hand-holding in order to agree to a CT scan, then that's simply one hour of staying later that day, one hour less of sleep, multiplied by an ever-growing roster of patients. Such math can't be helped. And in such a calculus, one less patient to argue with on a daily basis about dialysis is practically a gift!

I suppose the only way to work against such a utilitarian system is to periodically remind the residents—and myself—to stop for a moment in the day and subtract the other thirty-four patients from the list, so that there is just one patient there. How would we treat this patient if we had all the time in the world? What details might we address if we weren't barraged by unending tasks?

And then try to envision that problem patient as your mother, your grandfather, or, better yet, you. For that moment, imagine what it would like to be in that bed with those medical ailments saddled upon your body, and then see yourself as the physician walking into the room. How would you, the patient, react to you,

the doctor? The wisdom that you as the patient would offer...
perhaps that is the definition of compassion.

Ms. Binet resumed dialysis, but there was no panacea. The pain
management team gave her stronger pain meds, but these caused
more side effects. She required antibiotics for two more infections. The surgeons were furious that I had permitted Ms. Binet
to eat, and I had to defend my decision several times over. I also
had to gently—and repeatedly—remind them that I was the attending on the case and that they were the consultants.

Ms. Binet's medical conditions eventually reached a tenuous
equilibrium, enough that we could agree on a plan for her to go to
a short-term rehabilitation facility. I had doubts that she would
ever regain enough strength to return home, but she wanted that
option open to her, and this would be her best chance.

Kimberly and I spent the rest of the month in a strained relationship. Though she was sufficiently competent in her medical
skills, I found that I could not warm up to her. I thought back
to my PGY-II year and how unsettling it was to have clinical responsibilities yet still feel so close to the newness of internship.
To this day, the patients that I cared for at that awkward transition time are among the most vividly—and at times painfully—
remembered. I tried to be sympathetic to Kimberly's situation as
a PGY-II, but her businesslike efficiency always left me feeling
that we had missed something. I suppose there is no way to put
"compassion" on one's scut list, a task to be checked off when
completed.

Nor is it simple to teach. I hoped that working so closely together with patients would have been sufficient to share the skills
and values that are important. But in the end, it is the patient who
teaches this. I just wish I'd had the presence of mind to track Kimberly down when Ms. Binet's first meal tray arrived that evening.

Bellevue grub is not known for its culinary sophistication, but
food it is. Limp, lukewarm, perennially bland, but food. I myself
had only popped my head in the door for a moment to make sure
that her tray had arrived. Ms. Binet was still in her bed, but the head

had been raised to almost a sitting position. Her hands worked the plastic cutlery methodically and I imagined that she might be fantasizing about the robust fare from her native Salonika as she sawed through an entrée that I was unable to recognize. I waved from the door and she raised her fork in a small salute. She wasn't able to say anything though, because she was chewing, and she was obviously too polite to talk with her mouth full.

CHAPTER NINE

In Her Own Key

"Sorry to drag you down here at such a late hour. Can never tell when these chest pains will come, eh? Sure ruins a good vacation! I usually carry a letter from my doc up in Toronto with all my medicines and all the stuff that's ever happened to me. Course I didn't have it with me at the restaurant tonight when the pains started acting up. Janine went back to the hotel to get it out of my suitcase, because I know how much you doctors like those nice typed-up letters. Such a nice hotel; you guys really have nice hotels in this city."

She thrust a plump, freckled hand toward me and grinned. "Cheryl Holloway, but please, just call me Cheryl. Hate that 'Miss' stuff and I'm no 'Ms.'"

Twenty-nine years old with chest pain? She'd better give a good history. Two crummy minutes before midnight—they could've held this one for night float. Now I'm going to be here all night with this ridiculous chest pain.

Cheryl Holloway had just been moved from the ER to the CCU (cardiac care unit) where I was working in November of my second year of residency, the same point where Kimberly was when I would supervise her, years later, taking care of Marianne Binet. The PGY-II year of a medical residency—the middle year—is nearly universally recognized as the lowest, blackest portion of medical training. The nervous excitement of internship has worn off, the confidence and optimism of being a senior resident has yet to come. If the interns are the sweatshop laborers, the

PGY-IIs are the industry workhorses. They are responsible for a vast amount of medical care, yet they themselves are still making their way in the system. The intern is stuck putting in all the IVs and drawing endless tubes of blood, but it is the PGY-II who has to agonize over whether a patient is stable enough to survive the night or whether another medication or procedure should be done before going home. Caught between the sense that they are still defining themselves as doctors and the terror that their new-found responsibility will lead to death and mayhem, second-year residents often feel like they are churning in a vast black hole of despair.

Cheryl shoved a clump of red curly hair out of her eyes. Her left hand was curled around a can of ginger ale that she must have bought from one of the vending machines in the ER. A hospital-issue straw lolled about in the metal opening. Cheryl chattered on without much prompting from me. "Just about everybody in my family has heart problems. If you're a Holloway, you're gonna have a bad heart. That's what they say."

As she spoke, her right hand wandered to the metal bedside stand where someone had left a few stainless-steel clamps. She fiddled with them absentmindedly. "My sister and my aunt both had heart attacks when they weren't yet forty. I know that's the heritable type. I got diabetes and blood pressure too. They told me I had one of those silent heart attacks, but I never felt it. Had two of those balloon things. Last one 'bout a year ago."

Hmm, an angioplasty. Maybe there is something to her chest pain. But twenty-nine years old?

"They told me I had ninety percent stenosis of my right artery and fifty percent in my, what do they call that one, the obtuse something or other?"

Obtuse marginal artery. Half the medical students don't even know that artery.

"Good ejection fraction, though. Gotta be happy for that." She giggled, clinking the clamps together.

Maybe Ms. Holloway has one of those rare congenital heart dis-

eases. Could be kind of interesting. Maybe I'll present her case at our conference next week. But two friggin' minutes before midnight—I'll never make it home. Sometimes it feels like I live in Bellevue.

Last weekend I went to a concert at Carnegie Hall. I think it was my first time beyond the five-block radius of Bellevue in months. Probably my first time at Carnegie Hall since medical school graduation a year and a half ago.

"But the angioplasty," Cheryl continued, flipping the clamps over and letting them clomp against the metal tray, "what a weird thing. You ever have one, Doc? It's so weird to lie there awake on the table while they're fishing around in your heart. And you can see it all on the TV screens. Weird! This high-tech stuff is something else."

I swirled my ever-present cup of coffee to mix in the sugar. I'd already downed one cup and was hoping not to have to drink number three.

The nurse placed an EKG in my hands while Cheryl continued to toy with the clamps. The black heart tracings stood out against the background of finely printed pink graph paper. I ran my finger across the squiggles, hunting for any signs of a heart attack. The QRS complexes were bounding at a rate of over a hundred. I measured her PR interval and ST segments by counting out the tiny pink boxes with my fingernail—1 millimeter for every box long, 1 millivolt for every box high. I didn't see anything disastrous like ST-segment elevations or flipped T-waves. No sign of an acute MI, but with a heart rate that fast I couldn't rule out a heart attack with certainty.

Suddenly there was a cacophonous clatter as the bedside tray and the stainless-steel clamps upended onto the floor. "Ooh, sorry," Cheryl said, her hand snapping inward and coming to rest in her nest of curls. "I can be such a klutz, you know."

The clang echoed in my head, threatening to discombobulate any remaining shreds of organized thought. I closed my eyes instinctively in an attempt to stay focused, but the strident metallic sound continued to reverberate.

Cymbals, pretend it's cymbals instead of hemostat clamps. Cymbals in an orchestra, ringing out the climax. The symphony orchestra on stage in Carnegie Hall.

Cheryl reclined back in the bed that had been adjusted to a sitting-up position. "My other thing is that I get pyelo infection in my kidneys a lot. Like every six months. I'm always getting some kind of antibiotic or another—that's why I have no veins left! I've had every kind of central line: subclavians, jugulars, femorals. I've had Hickmans, PICC lines, Mediports, you name it! I tell you, residents sure get a lot of practice on me." Cheryl pulled down the neck of her gown and pointed out the marks from the various central intravenous lines. She flipped up her gown, revealing a fleshy white belly riddled with surgical scars.

"Don't forget the one in the back." She twisted around so I could see the three-inch surgical scar on her side. It was purplish and curved, with perpendicular crosshatches from the surgical staples that had been used to close it.

Cheryl crossed and uncrossed her legs under the sheets. "It's hard to get comfy in these beds, eh?" She took a sip of ginger ale. "These bendy straws are my favorite," she said. "Probably the best thing hospitals have to offer, don't you think?"

Cheryl pulled her knees up to her chest and curled her arms around them. "They finally had to put a tube inside one of my kidneys—one of them stents, or whatever you call it. What a pain in the butt that was! Still end up in the hospital once or twice a year, though. Can't ever seem to lick that pyelo. I can tell another episode is coming on now—that icky feeling in my side. And I been seeing some blood in my pee. That's what started the chest pains tonight. It always happens like that and I have to go back to Sick Kids for a week or two for antibiotics." She shrugged her shoulders and took another slurp of her soda.

Sick Kids, I know that name. Sick Kids. Where have I heard that before? That's the nickname for the Hospital for Sick Children in Toronto. See, it wasn't a total waste of time attending college in Canada. I bet no one else in Bellevue would've gotten that reference. That's not something the average hypochondriac would invent. I guess she is for real—but a pediatric hospital?

"I know what you're thinking, but the folks up at Sick Kids, they know me since I'm fourteen. They got all my records, so I still go there, even though I'm a little older now." She giggled with a conspiratorial wink. "I won't tell if you won't tell."

I flipped a clean sheet of paper onto my clipboard. Out of the corner of my eye I could see the CCU nurse leaning against the medication cabinet. She was one of those nurses who'd been at Bellevue for decades, but I could never remember her name. Her ID card dangled around her neck enmeshed in a swarm of keys, and it was invariably facing the wrong way. And I felt silly, anyway, staring down at her chest, squinting to read the microscopic print some idiot chose to use for the ID cards. And I'd already asked her at least seventeen times this year. I really did try to learn everyone's name, but there were so many nurses, and we residents got rotated every month. Was it Ms. Johnson? Or Miss Dellinger? It was too embarrassing to ask again.

I knew she was waiting for my admitting orders so she could get her work done—change of shift or assessment or something like that. Or maybe her break was coming up. I uncapped my pen and scribbled on the corner of a progress note, but the ink was fading. I fished in my pocket for another, but all I could come up with were my EKG calipers.

I turned toward the nurse and flashed a sheepish smile that I hoped looked sympathetic. She sighed and tossed me a pen from her pocket. Then she glanced at her blank order sheet.

"Sorry, Doctor, I should have carried my list of pills with me," Cheryl prattled on. "I know that wasn't too responsible of me, what with this bad heart and the diabetes and all. Janine should be back any minute now, but let me see what I can remember. I know most of them since I take them every day." She ticked the medications off on her fingers as she spoke. "There's the insulin—I take forty units in the morning, twenty-two units at night." I scribbled rapidly as she spoke. "For my heart I take labetalol and hydralazine, and of course an aspirin a day. Can't ever forget the aspirin, eh? My doctor told me a million times that aspirin was the most important pill for my heart. And for my blood pressure, let's see, there's the clonidine, and what's that other pill? Reserpine. Clonidine and reserpine."

My pen halted amid its rapid transcription of her words. *Reserpine? Who in their right mind ever prescribes reserpine? And clonidine is a fourth-line medication. So are hydralazine and labetalol. I know Canada has socialized medicine, but...*

Cheryl smiled and shrugged with a chuckle. "I know, I know, that combo sounds crazy. Every doctor gives me that look when they hear it, but I tell you, they tried everything else, and these are the only ones that work. Took years to finally get my pressure down. The doctors keep offering me these newfangled drugs, but I tell them I want to stay with what works: reserpine, hydralazine, labetalol, and clonidine. I'm not taking any chances with my health. Had enough problems already." She twisted her finger around one of her red curls and took another slurp of ginger ale.

Jeez, she must really have resistant hypertension... or crazy doctors. But it works—her BP is 130/85.

Do we even stock reserpine in the Bellevue pharmacy?

The nurse waved the blank order sheet at me. Her eyes traveled toward the clock on the wall and then back to me. 12:30 A.M.

Okay, I get your hint. Everybody wants the admitting orders the minute you've laid eyes on the patient. It takes time, you know, to take a history, do a physical exam, check the lab results, then come up with a diagnosis and plan. You can't just write orders without doing a careful evaluation, even if change of shift is coming up. Not every hear attack is the same. Give me a couple of minutes, will you?

I pressed my palms onto my forehead, trying to clear my brain to begin processing Cheryl Holloway's case.

It was an all-Beethoven night at Carnegie Hall. The orchestra was featuring the Sixth Symphony, my all-time favorite. I was eleven years old when I first heard it performed live. We were in Israel and Zubin Mehta was conducting an outdoor concert—my first concert ever. I watched Mehta raise his arms on that velvety summer night, and the bows of the stringed instruments responded in unison. It was magic—rows of violin and cello bows dancing together in a mellifluous ballet.

"Like I was saying, my aunt Tillie had a heart attack when she was thirty-seven. Shocked everybody that she passed away from it, because Tillie was so healthy."

Cheryl's voice jarred me back to the CCU. I hadn't realized that my mind was wandering and, obviously, neither had Cheryl.

"Tillie never ate a piece of red meat in her life. A health-food nut, she was. Listen, Doctor, I don't mean to bother you but I'm really in a lot of pain. This pyelo is killing me. Do you think you could give me something for the pain? Demerol is the one that works for my pyelo pain."

Something's fishy here. She doesn't look like she's in that much pain. But if she really has pyelonephritis...pyelo can be excruciatingly painful. I have to give her pain meds, even if it doesn't sit right with me. The ER note says they gave her fifty of Demerol a little while ago. Let's see if that holds her.

"I don't mean to be a nilly," Cheryl said, clasping her hands together, "but I've been through this so many times before. I know my body, Doctor. Fifty milligrams of Demerol never holds me. As you can see, I'm no skinny chicken." She patted her belly with a smile. "Fifty never does nothing to me. Maybe if I lost thirty pounds like my doctor is always bugging me to do, fifty milligrams of Demerol might lick that pyelo pain, but as it is, it probably just sits here in my fat. At Sick Kids, they always have to start me off with seventy-five."

She tugged at the ends of her hair, pulling the wiry locks almost straight. "I hate to be in this position, and I know you got more important stuff on your mind." She let the curls go and they sprang back into their tight amber helices.

I took another sip of coffee and swirled it around in my mouth. *Here it comes...a drug-seeker. I knew it. But is she making everything else up? She knows medical details that only someone who's been sick before would know. Something in her story is probably real, but I need to feel her out, get to know her better. Got to be careful with these drug-seekers, though; if you blow their confidence on the first round you'll never be able to get anything done. What's the big deal if I add another twenty-five? She is a bit on the hefty side, after all.*

She snapped up straight and her knees flattened out onto the bed as I loaded up the syringe. "It won't work if you just add twenty-five milligrams. It has to be seventy-five all at the same time. Please, Doctor, I've been through this a million times at Sick Kids. They had so much trouble with my pain that they had to get a special anesthesia doctor. Only seventy-five of Demerol works."

I've heard this routine before: they give you the sob story about the only medicine that works, then they plead and beg and annoy you until you prescribe it just to shut them up. She's not going to pull this one on me.

"The anesthesia doctor explained to me why it works that way," Cheryl said, staring up at me from the bed. Her pale hazel eyes were intermittently shadowed by the tickles of hair that swept by. "He said the loading dose, or something like that, has to be high enough, otherwise it won't ever work. If you don't load it, he said, you could be waiting till the cows come home to see any effect."

Well, maybe there is something with the absorption of the medication at different dosages.

The nurse rolled her eyes, still fingering the order sheet.

Don't give me that look. I don't know everything about every medicine; I'm still a PGY-II. I just need time to think, okay? There is a possibility, you know, that she's not a drug-seeker; I can't be absolutely sure. And pyelo can be very painful.

I swallowed another mouthful of coffee. I'd added two sugars but they did nothing to counteract the bitterness of the coffee. The cloying sweetness and the stale brininess coexisted defiantly, refusing to blend into a tolerable compromise.

I pulled another fifty milligrams into the syringe, closing one eye to read the total of seventy-five accurately.

I wish the nurse would stop giving me the evil eye. What does she expect me to do in this situation?

Come to think of it, that Zubin Mehta concert wasn't actually the very first time I'd heard the Sixth Symphony outdoors. It was the Disney film Fantasia *at the drive-in movie theater. I couldn't have been more than eight. I remember hooking the tiny portable speaker onto the edge of the car window. The familiar strains of Beethoven came through, if a bit scratchy, as the satyrs frolicked on the screen in their cartoon forest.*

"Let's see, where was I? My older sister, Sue, she got the blood pressure and diabetes like me. She been seeing the heart doctors since she was fifteen. Had an MI 'bout three or four years back. My aunt Tillie, my father's sister, died of a heart attack when she was thirty-seven. But I told you that, didn't I?"

The nurse sank into her chair and started doing her paperwork. But every few minutes she'd look up at me with that same annoyed expression. I knew I was holding things up for her and I wished I could make it go faster, but Cheryl Holloway was like a steamroller, and it was going to take some time to figure out which way was up and to avoid being flattened.

"And my father's brother, Uncle Arnold, he's got bad pressure and a couple of heart attacks. I guess he's in his sixties now, I don't know exactly, but seems he's always in the hospital for one thing or another. Can't walk much these days. My brother, Petey, he's okay, I guess. Got lucky, eh?"

That's some set of genes she's walking around with ... if she's telling the truth. But why wouldn't she? This would be a lot of stuff to invent. And who the hell would ever know about reserpine or the obtuse marginal artery? And she did get a cardiac angiogram. If it's all true, I can't blow off her chest pain story.

I scrawled a family tree on my page: circles for girls, squares for boys, colored-in for heart disease, diagonal slashes for deaths. It wasn't a pretty picture.

The nurse came over with a cup for a urine sample.

"Just a minute," Cheryl snapped. "Can't you see I'm talking with the doctor? I'll pee when I'm good and ready! How do you expect anyone to pee around here with all this pressure? Talk about manners."

She turned to me and smiled. "I know, I know. You want to see if there's blood in my urine from the pyelo. By now I certainly know that one: blood in the pee equals pyelo. I tell you, I should go to medical school already. I have the experience, eh? But I can't pee when the nurses keep bugging me. I have shy kidneys, you know? Now where was I?"

Okay, okay, I get the picture. Just shut up already and let me do the physical exam. If I don't do the physical, I'll never get the admitting note finished. And if I don't get the admitting orders written I'm going to have this nurse on my case all night. And I have to present that lupus case at Morning Report tomorrow and I still haven't rounded up all the X-rays. And tomorrow's Tuesday so I have clinic all afternoon. By the time I get all my work done tomorrow it'll be midnight again.

I chugged back the last of my coffee and got a coppery swig of undissolved sugar and coffee-ground scum.

"Now, what was I saying? My father, right. He's got high pressure like everybody else, and my ma is always trying to get him to stick to his diet. He's got bad cholesterol. He talks about chest pains and stuff, but I don't know if he's ever had a real heart attack, unless he's had the silent type, like me. He used to work down at Petro-Canada, but he can't do that no more. He had to retire on account of his heart. We're some family, eh? When Janine gets here with my doctor's letter, you'll get the whole story."

All right, everyone in your family has heart disease. Your dog has heart disease. Let me do my physical exam and write my admitting note so I can get out of this place before the sun rises.

"I don't know what's taking Janine so long anyway. The hotel is in midtown, right near that skyscraper. The one with all the lights—you know which one I'm talking about, right? It has a bar way up on the top floor. You can see the whole damn world from there—pardon my French."

I ran my stethoscope along Cheryl's chest and she obliged me by taking deep breaths without my even asking, but she continued talking. Her words rebounded in her chest and echoed through my stethoscope. "And I said to Janine, 'You know, Janine, when you're up this high in Manhattan with a piña colada in your hand, you know you've made it.' No joking, that's what I said to her."

ADMITTING DIAGNOSES:

1 MI vs. unstable angina in patient with strong medical history, though EKG without signs of cardiac disease
 • *admit to CCU for cardiac monitoring*
 • *continue labetalol, reserpine, clonidine, and hydralazine*
 • *consider switching to more current meds*

2 Hypertension
 • *takes unusual meds, but BP well controlled*

3 Acute pyelonephritis
 • *check urine for blood, bacteria, and white cells*
 • *begin IV antibiotics, pain meds as needed*

4 Diabetes
 • *check blood and urine for glucose*
 • *continue current insulin regimen*

Should I add "possible drug addiction"? The attendings, though, are always telling us to watch what we write. "The chart is a legal document; be careful what you write down," they always say. I can't just put down my gut feelings, it wouldn't be fair to the patient. And who knows, maybe ten years from now, someone will pull out this chart and sue me for defamation.

But the way she asks for Demerol—with that 75/25 business—there's something that makes me queasy. Dr. Jones used to tell us to pay attention to what we were feeling during the interview. It was my first year of med school. "Patients with depression make you feel depressed," she said. "Patients with anxiety get you anxious." Well, what about patients who just give you the heebie-jeebies?

Cheryl watched me as I wrote out her CCU admitting orders. She followed my hand as I turned the page to complete the diagnosis and medication allergy section. When I looked up for a second to calculate the IV flow rate, her hazel eyes were fixed on mine. And her finger never stopped twisting a red curl.

"Listen, Doc, I appreciate everything you're doing for me," Cheryl said. "I know you have a lot of work to do—I been in the CCU before—but I hope you order the Demerol q one hour because this pyelo is like the devil. It's even worse than the chest pains. Once the antibiotics start working I know the pain will go away, but till they kick in, it could be a while."

Q one hour? Is she crazy? It's a q-four-hour medication! Nobody gets Demerol every hour; that much I know for sure. I'm not going to be a narcotics dispensary for this little tart. Even if she is having the worst pyelonephritis in the world.

I slammed the cap back on my pen but missed and sank a line of black ink down my right hand.

But what's the point of trying to keep a drug addict off drugs? It's not going to work and I'm the one who's going to suffer. I should just give her all the Demerol she wants and then go to bed. Then both she and I will get some sleep.

The ink had settled into the creases of my palm. I tore open an alcohol swab and started rubbing. The black ink spread into a grayish blotch.

Cheap drug company pens.

But I can't just give out narcotics to an addict. I don't want to be abetting someone's drug habit. What if she overdoses? And she could still have heart disease in addition to being a drug addict. Cocaine can even cause heart attacks by itself. Her EKG shows only sinus tach, but the rapid heart rate could mask the signs of a heart attack.

I wiped my hand on my lab coat to get rid of the cold alcohol, and the gray smeared onto the white.

But I couldn't possibly order q-one-hour Demerol, could I? That nurse will think I'm totally incompetent, which she probably already does. But technically a doctor is allowed to order a drug any way they want.

And what about Quality Assurance, or Quality Control, or whatever that office is? I've heard they pick through the charts with a fine-toothed comb. Administering narcotics at four times the recommended frequency...that'll get me some attention. I'm not messing with this stuff. Forget about it.

"You can so do it! That's how they do it at Sick Kids. It's q one hour!"

Sick Kids. Enough with the Sick Kids. This is Bellevue. We don't prescribe a q-four-hour drug for every hour.

"Please don't do this to me, Doctor." Cheryl's voice thinned out and started to crack. "It never lasts four hours. I'm so afraid of the pain."

No, don't start whining. Please.

Cheryl pursed her lips together, but I could see they were starting to quiver. "This pyelo aches so much. It's like a fire that just burns from the inside out." Her freckles were trembling and she started to sniffle. "This is the way it always happens. I try to take just a little vacation and end up in the ER. This is the price I pay. Is it too much to ask in this world to have a little vacation without getting sick?"

The entranceway to Carnegie Hall was glistening. The gold leaf on the ceiling and the shimmering lights. The sounds of rustling silk and pattering heels. The crisp, inky smell of freshly printed pro-

grams. The snippets of conversation about theater, art, and poli-
tics. The air was charged as people scurried to their seats, gulping
the last of their chardonnay. The orchestra was warming up and
I could hear familiar phrases trickling out in random order like a
jazz improv session.

The nurse swiveled in her chair to face me. She folded her arms
across her chest once again, upsetting the collection of keys that
hung around her neck. Twenty years of Bellevue experience was
what that look was saying to me. Twenty years.

"Every time I get pyelo, it's always like this," Cheryl wept.
There was a supply bin overhead and I plunged my hand in,
scrambling around for a box of tissues. Three rolls of surgical tape
tumbled to the floor. "Nobody ever believes me. The pyelo gets
worse and worse until it sets off the chest pains." She thrust her
hands in her lap and hung her head down. Her shock of red curls
spilled over her face. "I'm going to end up like my aunt Tillie: dead
at thirty-seven from the Holloway heart."

Don't make me feel like an ogre for refusing a request for pain
meds. I can't take it when they start to cry. I'm never going to win
with this lady. Maybe I'll write an as-needed order for every two
hours.

The nurse pulled the string of keys off her neck and slapped it
onto the desk. She flipped the keys through her fingers one by one
as I wrote the order. Each one turned over with a resounding
clank. Twenty years.

Leave me alone. I don't need it from you also. You're supposed
to be on my side.

"No, not p.r.n., please," Cheryl said, grabbing for my sleeve.
"Please, Doctor, don't leave me in pain. I've had so much experience in hospitals." Her sobs grew ragged as she gulped in tight,
anxious breaths. "If it's p.r.n. I have to wait so long to get the meds.
You residents work so hard. I know you have a tough schedule
and it takes so long for you to come each time the nurse calls you.
It would just be easier if you wrote a q-one-hour *standing* order
so it will be there for me when I need it." She tugged my arm to-

ward her. "I know my body, Doctor. Please don't make me suffer like this."

The nurse mouthed *Don't you dare* at me.

The oboe sang out its A note — delicate and plaintive. The other musicians paused to listen, then they tuned their instruments to match. The cacophony evened out to one single, echoing note that swept across the stage, out to the audience, up over the balconies, gathering the length and breadth of the concert hall in its pure-toned embrace.

"I can't take the pain anymore," Cheryl whimpered. "Please, Doctor, I don't know who else to turn to. I have no family here. Please don't make me suffer."

Cheryl pulled the blankets high up over her chin. All I could see now was her red hair, eyebrows, and the top of her nose. There was an arc of freckles across her forehead. She'd closed her eyes, but there were tears seeping out from under her delicate blond eyelashes.

But what if I withhold? What if I miss that single person in the sea of manipulative drug users who really is in pain? What if one person remains in agony because I didn't believe their words? Ms. Twenty-Years-at-Bellevue doesn't have to live with the decision. I'm sure she hates to be the one who actually administers the medicines to these addicts, but she doesn't have to live with the decision. Maybe I'll order a lower dose of morphine, just so there's something every hour to keep this patient quiet.

"Thank you, Doctor. You're really saving my life." Cheryl clasped my hand to her heart. "I think you have a special calling to medicine. It's a gift from God to be able to help people. You are truly blessed."

She turned toward the nurse and hollered, "Can I get the first dose now?"

The nurse slammed her keys on the desk. They echoed with a harsh metallic thud. She held up the Demerol bottle from which I'd given Cheryl seventy-five milligrams half an hour ago.

"That was Demerol!" Cheryl snapped. "It doesn't count. The

morphine is for breakthrough pain, and I'm having breakthrough pain. Can't you see that the doctor is writing a separate order for morphine? Are you going to let me sit here and suffer?"

The nurse swept her keys off the desk and marched over to the supply cabinet. She started taking inventory of the endotracheal tubes, slapping them on the counter one by one.

The orchestra finished their tuning and sat waiting. The conductor strode on stage in his sleek black coat.

"Well, tell this damn nurse to stop pestering me. She has no idea what it's like to be a patient. She's never had pyelonephritis or chest pains. When Janine gets here, you'll see my whole history. It's got the doses of the pain meds and everything. My doctor told me to always carry that letter with me." She sniffled and rubbed a lock of hair against her eyelid to catch a newly budding tear. "Nobody ever believes me. You just don't know what it's like to hurt so much."

She's right. I don't know what it's like to hurt so much. I've never been that sick before and I've never been in a position where someone else has control over what happens to my body. If she were sixty years old, I wouldn't even think twice, but heart attacks and hypertension don't typically occur in a twenty-nine-year-old. But maybe Cheryl Holloway is that one exception.

> **CCU PROGRESS NOTE:** called by RN multiple times in past hour for pain meds. Patient verbally abusive to RN. Patient also complaining of chest pain, but EKG shows only sinus tach. Chest pain not responsive to sublingual nitroglycerin, only to Demerol and morphine.

The nurse pulled me aside and warned me that I'd better "do something" about "my patient." Otherwise, there might be an incident report.

Do something? What am I supposed to do? Transform her into another personality? Tie her down and stuff a sock in her mouth? And she's not my patient. I didn't invite her to Bellevue to make your life miserable. Do you think I'm enjoying myself? Two damn minutes before midnight. This all could've been night float's responsibility.

"That bitch won't give me my medicine." Cheryl spat toward the nurse. "I am very sick. I need my medicine." The nurse glared at me and reached for the telephone.

This is all I need now. I can't afford to have a bad relationship with this nurse, otherwise my whole year will be miserable. These lifetime nurses at Bellevue know how to torture you if they want. You can't cross 'em.

"You nurses are all alike," Cheryl hollered. "You don't give a damn that I'm in pain. You just love to make patients suffer. All you care about is getting your damn coffee break every four hours. You never took no Hippocratic Oath. Only the doctors really care about your pain."

The nurse turned away and stared at the opposite wall. Her fingers dialed the phone without her even having to look at the numbers.

Cheryl sniffled and slurped the last of her soda out of the can she'd been holding for the past hour. "My doctor at Sick Kids was the most devoted man I've ever met," she whimpered. "He was just like you, working all night without sleep. But he always managed to stop by before he went home. He made sure I had all the right medicines. When he was taking care of me I never had any pain."

I could see the nurse consulting with her supervisor. Their huddled bodies under the doorframe blocked the light from the hallway.

Great. Go over my head to your supervisor. That's really helpful. Maybe this lady is just an addict, but she did come in complaining of chest pain and gave a history of significant coronary disease. I have to take her word and treat her. Even if she is annoying, and even if she is also a drug addict, I still have to treat her. If I didn't it would be malpractice. And unethical. It's not my job to make everyone play nice—they didn't teach us any of that in medical school—I'm just trying to make sure she's not having pyelonephritis or a heart attack.

"This pyelo is killing me," Cheryl said, her face puckering up with tears. "My kidneys are acting up. I know there is an infection, I can just feel it." She thrust a specimen cup into my hand. "Look at all the blood in my urine."

Uggh, that certainly is a lot of blood. I hate it when they hand me specimens before I get a chance to put gloves on. I know the cover is screwed on, but still...

That's a real blood clot in there. Pyelo doesn't usually present with clots—it presents with microscopic blood. How did she get a blood clot in there? She has had multiple episodes of pyelonephritis before and has an internal kidney stent. Maybe that could cause a clot. But clot or no clot, if she's diabetic I can't take any chances with an infection. It could spread to her whole body in a few hours. She has to get IV antibiotics immediately, at least until the urine culture results come back in twenty-four hours.

The nurse had returned from her doorway consultation and was now taking Cheryl's vital signs. She refused to make eye contact with me.

"I don't have to cooperate with nobody," Cheryl was saying while the nurse slipped the blood pressure cuff around her arm. "I'm the patient. I'm sick. I have to get my medicines! Get this bitch away from me." She whisked her arm back, disconnecting the cuff from its cord. The nurse grabbed for the cuff and Cheryl swatted at her to keep her away.

The conductor raised his hands high, his baton aloft. The violin bows swung upward in unison, poised to begin. He held the musicians at attention until there was a spell of complete silence in all of Carnegie Hall. I held my breath, hanging on to the tense stillness, savoring the anticipation.

"This fuckin' hospital sucks! You people don't have a clue what you're doing. At Sick Kids they know how to take care of me. That's a real academic hospital. This place is just a stupid city hospital." A large glob of spit sailed across the room.

CCU PROGRESS NOTE: Patient spitting at RN and physically threatening. RN requesting order for restraints.

Listen, I'm pretty damn proud of Bellevue. Sick Kids probably has twice the budget of Bellevue. Just because they have fancier MRIs and nicer furniture doesn't mean they're a better hospital.

The nurse and her supervisor swiftly secured Cheryl's wrists to the railings with white cloth ties. "Get the hell off me, you witches. I'm a Canadian citizen." Her voice lowered to a growl. "You can't hold me prisoner here. I know my rights." The nurse and the night supervisor quickly pulled back to get out of spitting range.

The first notes of the Sixth Symphony rose from the orchestra—gentle, almost too soft to hear. The phrase was simple and unadorned, the violins climbing up and over an F-major chord. Then they paused, leaving the phrase as a question, an invitation. The cellos and violas answered, repeating back the motif an octave lower. But before they could finish the entire phrase, the violin sections slipped back in. Slowly at first, then with greater urgency, filling out the melody with a breathtaking lushness. All the bows of all the strings were dancing together, gliding in a lissome waltz.

"Get me out of this goddamn place. Untie me and let me out. Now!" Red, curly hair flew about as Cheryl twisted her head violently, trying to shake off the restraints. "I know about the Geneva Convention. I could bring charges against you. Let me go back to Canada, where they treat you like a human being."

She wants to leave; that's the best news I've heard all night. My head is about to split open and this nurse is either going to strangle me with her stethoscope or have me written up by that supervisor. All I want to do is go home and put Beethoven's Sixth Symphony on my stereo. Well, maybe a hot shower first, and some breakfast. But then I want to sit on my couch—perfectly still—and listen to the music. I don't want to think about anything else. I just want to sit there and listen to Beethoven. All nine symphonies in a row. That's all I want in this life: nine symphonies without being paged or spit at. Is that too much to ask?

"Get me out of here," Cheryl yelled through her gnashing teeth. "I can sue you for this. My cousin is a lawyer. An international lawyer!"

> **CCU PROGRESS NOTE:** Patient requesting to leave against medical advice. Medical condition unclear: lab results and X-rays still pending.

But what if she really does have cardiac disease? Everything she's said makes some sense, not like the regular Bellevue addicts who dish out the lamest stories to get drugs. I can't say for sure that this is not *a heart attack in progress.*

"That nurse has it out for me." A small arc of spit landed on the floor. "I demand to talk to the head of the hospital. That bitch won't give me the medicines I need. That's in the Geneva Convention also. They should fire her for malpractice."

And does she truly possess decisional capacity to leave the hospital with a potentially life-threatening condition? This is a public hospital and our patients aren't quite as litigious as those folks at the private hospitals, but what if she's the one patient who has a cardiac arrest right out on First Avenue?

"You Yankee assholes can't keep me here against my will; I'm a Canadian citizen. My father knows the ambassador." I reached down to check her pulse. Her plump wrist was largely covered by the restraints so I had to fish around under the cloth to find the skittering thump. Her teeth snapped toward my hand; I pulled back just in time.

If I open that can of worms, though, we'll be here all night waiting for the psychiatry consult to show up. I could just sign the papers myself; she'd be out of here in five minutes and I'd be asleep in a jiffy. I mean, there's no one here but me and the nurse. All I have to do is witness her signature saying that she understands the risks of leaving. She'll be out of my hair, the nurse will stop torturing me, I won't have to do all the admission paperwork, and I might even get to listen to that symphony before I qualify for Social Security.

"Untie me, you bastards." Her voice was more muffled now, but still audible, through the orange surgical mask the nurse had tied over her mouth. "Get me the fuck out of here. I'm a Canadian citizen. I have my rights."

But how can I say that a screaming, spitting, vicious patient clearly understands the risks of refusing treatment? If she has pyelonephritis and doesn't receive antibiotics, the infection could spread to her bloodstream. If she's having a heart attack and doesn't get treated she could potentially die. The right thing is to get a psych eval. But the nurse is going to hate me.

"A shrink? I ain't talking to no shrink. Get me the police." Cheryl's voice pitched upward and shrieked through the mask. "I'm going to file a malpractice suit against you. You're going to be responsible for my pyelo infection spreading and my heart attack. My cousin is a lawyer, you know."

The strings pulled back, leaving just the first violins to carry the melody. And then, right there in the middle of the phrase, without any pause, the melody was entrusted to a single flute. Just one flute in the vast expanse of Carnegie Hall carrying the motif. One silver flute singing out. Thousands of human beings pinned to their red velvet seats by the power of one instrument. One delicate melody holding up the roof, supporting the walls, balancing the balconies. One simple musical phrase arresting humanity dead in its tracks.

I paged the psych consult for an emergent evaluation. While I was on the phone the nurse sat at her desk looking from the clock over to Cheryl, then back to the clock. 2:00 A.M. The discharge papers were in her hand, and I knew she just wanted me to sign them without wasting time on psych.

After two long, loud hours the psychiatry resident finally

showed up. I could hear the conversation from the other side of the curtain.

"It's a pleasure to make your acquaintance, Dr. Levy," Cheryl chirped sweetly. "Yes, I'm down visiting from Toronto and my pyelo acted up again. Then I got the chest pains, right in the middle of this midtown restaurant. I didn't even get to finish the appetizer—those big, fancy mushrooms all sliced up like a deck of cards. You know the kind I'm talking about. And the waiters were so nice, trying to help and all. Who says New Yorkers aren't friendly?"

I sat at the clerk's desk at 4:30 A.M. writing Cheryl's discharge papers after the psychiatrist left. The nurse was positioned at the opposite desk charting the vital signs. Her keys dangled over the page where she was writing and she didn't once look up at me.

Come on, don't be so mad at me. I'm not trying to make your life difficult; I'm just trying to do the right thing. If I'd known that the psychiatrist was going to declare her competent, then I wouldn't have wasted everybody's time. But I wasn't sure. I know that you've been at Bellevue forever and you've seen every trick in the book, but I wasn't sure. I'm still a PGY-II. I guess that in your eyes I'm just another one of the hordes of residents who pass through here—giving orders like the captain of some ship but green as an Irish meadow. I can't help the way things are set up around here. I can only try to do my best.

I placed the pen that I'd borrowed earlier on the desk where she was sitting. She paused for a minute from her writing and her eyes slipped over to my ID card to look at my name. I could see the fatigue weighing down the corners of her eyes.

"I'll take care of removing the central line," I said. "I know you have a lot of work to do."

"Fine. Take your stupid central line out," Cheryl snapped when I walked over to her. "Just get me the hell out of here and away from you fucking doctors."

Okay, just clip the stitches and ease the central line out, nice and slow. Just like you'd do with a rabid dog—nice and slow, no sudden moves. Compress the bleeding site on her thigh. Act calm, don't say anything that might set her off.

"When I get back home I'm going to file a lawsuit like you Yanks ain't never seen before," Cheryl said. "You'd better start getting your lousy greenbacks together in a pile, because you'll be hearing from my lawyer real soon."

The flute continued to sing and then pulled in the oboes, then the clarinets, then the bassoons. The strings eased in quietly and so did the brass and before you could exhale, the entire orchestra was in a furious fortissimo that spun through the hall, bouncing off the tiers, giving you an exhilarating vertigo.

I pressed one hand onto her thigh to staunch the bleeding, and with the other, I curled the central line into garbage.

As soon as this bleeding stops I can leave here. Don't think about this crazy patient and the fact that she might bite you. Stay focused on the maestro's baton coaxing that intoxicating music from the mortals seated onstage, the humans equipped with nothing more than pieces of wood and metal. Watch them sweat as they stride their way toward the finale, arms flying, mouths blowing, fingers running, bows dancing. The music has spun around your head so that you don't know what direction it's coming from anymore, but it doesn't matter. It's coming from every direction and gravity has ceased to be an issue and you've been swept out of your seat, floating, swirling in a sea of music until the final gargantuan note slams you against the back of your seat.

And then you open your eyes, not quite sure where you are, but not particularly caring because you've woken up in bliss and Bellevue doesn't exist and there are no patients and no beepers and no sickness and no death. Just the gasp that shudders through your system as you settle into a deep peace and you are so alive.

CCU PROGRESS NOTE: Patient signed AMA discharge form and left without further incident.

I watched Cheryl Holloway march out the door, her red curls coiling ferociously with each stride. "I'm going to sue all you incompetent fucking bastards when I get home. My cousin is a lawyer, you know."

I slumped over on the desk with my head in my arms. I couldn't believe she was actually gone. I closed my eyes, listening to the sudden silence. Her dissonant voice was finally gone and my ears could relax. She was probably already heading to another ER to sing her song again. I couldn't decide if I should feel pity for Cheryl Holloway or anger for her pilfering of my precious night of sleep. It didn't really matter at this point; it was almost morning and I had to present that lupus case at Morning Report. I still hadn't tracked down all the X-rays.

There was a plunk next to my head and I raised my eyelids in its direction. It was a cup of coffee. "They just made a fresh pot in the lounge," the nurse said. "You look like you need a dose."

CCU NOTE, POSTDISCHARGE ADDENDUM:

Cardiac enzymes: within normal limits.

Blood glucose: normal.

Cholesterol: normal.

Urine: no glucose, white cells, or bacteria.

Abdominal X-ray: within normal limits, no kidney stent seen.

Final diagnosis: Probable Munchausen's Syndrome with deliberately induced sickness to obtain medical attention.

CHAPTER TEN

SAT

"NEMESIO RIOS?" I CALLED OUT to the crowded waiting room of our medical clinic. I'd just finished a long stint attending on the wards and I was glad to be back to the relatively sane life of the clinic. "Nemesio Rios?" I called out again.

"Yuh," came a grunt, as a teenaged boy in baggy jeans with a ski hat pulled low over his brow hoisted himself up. He sauntered into my office and slumped into the plastic chair next to my desk.

"What brings you to the clinic today?"

He shrugged. "Feel all right, but they told me to come today," he said, slouching lower into the chair, his oversize sweatshirt reaching nearly to his knees. The chart said he'd been in the ER two weeks ago for a cough.

"How about a regular checkup?" He shrugged again. His eyes were a rich brown, tucked deep beneath his brow.

Past medical history? None. Past surgical history? None. Meds? None. Allergies? None. Family history? None.

"Where were you born?" I asked, wanting to know his nationality.

"Here."

"Here in New York?"

"Yeah, in this hospital."

"A Bellevue baby!" I said with a grin, noticing that his medical record number had only six digits (current numbers had nine digits). "A genuine Bellevue baby."

There was a small smile, but I could see him working hard to suppress it. "My mom's from Mexico."

"Have you ever been there?" I asked, curious.

"You sound like my mom." He rolled his eyes. "She's always trying to get me to go. She's over there right now visiting her sisters."

"You don't want to go visit?"

"Mexico? Just a bunch of corrupt politicians." Nemesio shifted his unlaced sneakers back and forth on the linoleum floor, causing a dull screech each time.

I asked about his family. In a distracted voice, as though he'd been through this a million times before, he told me that he was the youngest of eight, but now that his sister got married, it was only he and his mother left in East Harlem. I asked about his father.

"He lives in Brooklyn." Nemesio poked his hand in and out of the pocket of his sweatshirt. "He's all right, I guess, but he drinks a lot," he said, his voice trailing off. "Doesn't do anything stupid, but he drinks."

"Are you in school now?"

"Me?" he said, his voice perking up for the first time from his baseline mumble. "I'm twenty. I'm done! Graduated last year."

"What are you doing now?"

"Working in a kitchen. It's all right, I guess."

"Any thoughts about college?"

"You sound like my cousin in Connecticut. He's in some college there and he's always bugging me about going to college. But I'm lazy. No one to kick my lazy butt."

"What do you want to do when you grow up?"

"What I *really* want to do? I want to play basketball." He gave a small laugh. "But they don't take five-foot-seven guys in the NBA."

"Anything else besides basketball?"

He thought for a minute. "Comics. I like to draw comics. I guess I could be an artist that draws comics." His eye caught the tiny Monet poster I'd taped above the examining table. "That's pretty cool, that painting."

"There are a lot of great art schools here in New York." My comment floated off into empty space. We were silent for a few minutes. I made a few notes in the chart.

"That stuff about peer pressure is a bunch of shit," he said abruptly, forcefully, sitting up in his chair, speaking directly toward the poster in front of him.

I leaned closer toward Nemesio, trying to figure out what this sudden outburst was related to. But he continued, staring straight forward, lecturing at the empty room, as if I weren't there.

"Anyone who tells you they do something because of peer pressure is full of shit." He was even more animated now, even angry. "People always asking me to do stuff, but I can make my own mind up." His hands came out of his sweatshirt pocket and began gesticulating in the air. "My brother and his friends, they're always drinking beer. But I don't like the taste of it. I don't believe in peer pressure."

Speech ended, Nemesio settled back into his chair, resumed his slouched posture, and repositioned his hands into his pockets. Then he glanced up at the ceiling and added quietly, almost wistfully, "But if beer tasted like apple juice, I might be drinking it every day."

He was quiet for a few minutes. One hand slid out of his pocket and started fiddling with the zipper on his sweatshirt.

Without warning he swiveled in his chair to face me directly, his whole body leaning into my desk. "You ever face peer pressure, Doc?"

His eyes were right on mine, and I was caught off guard by this sudden shift in his voice and body language. I felt unexpectedly on the spot. Who does he see? I wondered. Do I represent the older generation or the medical profession or women or non-Hispanic whites? Or all of the above?

Nemesio refused to let my gaze wander off his. He demanded

an answer to his question, and our doctor-patient encounter had obviously taken an abrupt turn. I could tell that a lot was riding on my answer, though I wasn't sure what exactly was at stake. Did he need me to provide a reassuring societal answer about how bad drugs are? Or did he need me to identify with him, to say that I've been where he's been, even if that was not exactly the truth?

"Yes," I said, after debating in my head for a moment, trying to think of something sufficiently potent to satisfy the question but not so sordid as to embarrass myself. "I have."

He stared at me, waiting for me to continue. His eyes looked younger and younger.

"In my first year of college," I said. "In the very first week. Everyone was sitting in the stairwell and they were passing a joint around. Everyone took a drag. When it came to me I hesitated. I wasn't really interested in smoking, but everyone else was doing it."

"So what did you do?"

"I didn't want anyone to think I was a little kid, so I took a drag too."

"Did you like it?"

"No, I just hacked and coughed. I didn't even *want* the stupid joint to begin with, and I couldn't believe I was doing it just because everyone else was."

"That peer pressure is shit." Nemesio stated it as a fact and then sank back into his seat.

"You're right. It is. It took me a little while to figure that out."

He pushed the ski hat back from his brow a few inches. "In my high school there was this teacher that was always on my case. She was always bugging me to study and take the tests. What a pain in the butt she was." He pulled the hat all the way off. "But now there's no one around to kick my lazy butt. I could get to college easy, but I'm just lazy."

My mind wandered back to a crisp autumn day in my second month of medical school. Still overwhelmed by the pentose-phosphate shunt and other minutiae of biochemistry, our Clinical Correlation group—led by two fourth-year students—promised us first-year students a taste of clinical medicine.

The CC student leaders had obtained permission for a tour of the New York City medical examiner's office. All suspicious death—murders, suicides, and the like—were investigated here.

The autumn sun dazzled against the bright turquoise bricks of the ME building, which stood out in sharp contrast to the gray concrete buildings lining First Avenue. We congregated on the steps, endeavoring to look nonchalant.

The security guard checked our ID cards as well as our letter of entry. We followed him through the metal detector, down the whitewashed concrete hallway, into the unpainted service elevator with a hand-pulled metal grate.

We stared at our sneakers as the elevator lurched downward. It creaked past several floors and landed with a jolt. Out we spilled, gingerly, onto the raw concrete floor. Our first stop was the morgue. The cavernous walk-in refrigerator was icy and silent. There was a Freon smell, the kind I recalled from the frozen food departments in grocery stores. As a child, when I went shopping with my mother I used to lean into the bins of ice cream and frozen waffles and inhale that curiously appealing, vaguely sweet, chemical fragrance. But here the odor was intensified—magnified by the rigid chill and bleak soundlessness of the room.

Nine naked corpses lay on shelves, their wizened bodies covered with skin that glowed a ghastly green from the low-wattage fluorescent lights. These were the unclaimed bodies, mostly elderly men found on the streets. The ones that were never identified, never claimed by relatives. The ones that were sent next door to the medical school. These were the subjects of our first-year anatomy course.

From there we were herded into the autopsy room. Loosely swinging doors delivered us into a shock of cacophonous noise and harsh bright lights. We stumbled into each other, a discombobulated mass at the entranceway, blinking to adjust from the stark silence of the morgue. The autopsy room was long and rectangular. The high ceilings and brisk yellow walls lent an odd air of cheeriness. Seven metal tables lay parallel in the center. Six of them were surrounded by groups of pathology residents performing autopsies. The residents wore long rubber gloves and industrial-strength aprons. The sound of their voices and their clanking instruments echoed in the room.

The only body I had ever opened was my cadaver in anatomy lab, which was preserved in formaldehyde and completely dried out. I'd never actually seen blood. In the autopsy room there was blood everywhere. Residents were handling organs—weighing hearts, measuring kidneys, taking samples from livers—then replacing them in the open corpses. Their aprons were spotted with scarlet streaks. Blood streamed down the troughs that surrounded each table.

It was disgusting, but I wasn't nauseated. These bodies didn't look like people anymore. It was more like a cattle slaughterhouse: cows and pigs lined up to be transformed into sterile packages of cellophane-wrapped chopped meat. The slaughterhouse that compelled you to vow lifetime vegetarianism, a resolve that lasted only until the next barbecue with succulent, browned burgers that looked nothing like the disemboweled carcasses you'd seen earlier.

Then I spied the last table, the only one without a sea of activity around it. Lying on the metal table was a young boy who didn't look older than twelve. He was wearing new Nikes and one leg of his jeans was rolled up to the knee. His bright red basketball jersey was pushed up, revealing a smooth brown chest. He looked as if he were sleeping.

I tiptoed closer. Could he really be dead? There was not a mark on his body. Every part was in its place. His clothes were crisp and clean. There was no blood, no dirt, no sign of struggle. He wasn't anything like the gutted carcasses on the other tables. His expression was serene, his face without blemish. His skin was plump. He was just a beautiful boy sleeping.

I wanted to rouse him, to tell him to get out of this house of death, quick, before the rubber-aproned doctors got to him. There is still time, I wanted to say. Get out while you can!

I leaned over his slender, exposed, adolescent chest. I peered closer. There, just over his left nipple, was a barely perceptible hole. Smaller than the tip of my little finger. A tiny bullet hole.

I stared at that hole. That ignominious hole. That hole that stole this boy's life. I wanted to rewind the tape, to give him a chance to dodge six inches to the right. That's all he'd need—just six inches. Who would balk over six inches?

Somebody pulled on my arm. Time to go.

For months after my visit to the medical examiner's office, I had nightmares. But they weren't about bloody autopsies or refrigerated corpses. I dreamt only about the boy, that beautiful, untouched, intact boy. The one who'd had the misfortune to fall asleep in the autopsy room.

At night, he would creep into my bed. On the street, I could feel his breath on the back of my neck. In the library, while I battled the Krebs cycle and the branches of the trigeminal nerve, he would slip silently into the pages of my book. His body was so perfect, so untouched.

Except for that barely perceptible hole.

———

Now I looked at Nemesio Rios sitting before me; his beautiful body adrift in the uncertainty of adolescence, made all the rockier by the unfair burdens of urban poverty. Research has shown that health status and life expectancy are directly correlated with socioeconomic status and earning power. Whether this is related to having health insurance, or simply to having more knowledge to make healthier lifestyle choices, there is no doubt that being poor is bad for your health.

As I scribbled in his chart, an odd thought dawned on me: the best thing that I, as a physician, could recommend for Nemesio's long-term health would be to take the SAT and get into college. Too bad I couldn't just write a prescription for that.

"Have you taken the SAT yet?" I asked Nemesio.

"Nah. I can't stand U.S. history. What's the point of knowing U.S. history?"

I twisted my stethoscope around my finger. "Ever hear of McCarthy?"

He shrugged. "Yeah, maybe."

"McCarthy tried to intimidate people to turn in their friends and coworkers. Anyone who might believe differently from him. I'd hate to see that part of U.S. history repeated."

He nodded slowly. "Yeah, I guess. I wouldn't want nobody to tell me what to think. That peer pressure is shit."

"Besides," I added, "there's no U.S. history on the SAT."

Nemesio turned toward me, his eyes opened wide. "Yeah? No U.S. history?" His cheeks were practically glowing.

"No history. Just math and English."

"Wow," he said. "No U.S. history. That's pretty cool." His tone of voice changed abruptly as his gaze plummeted to the floor. "But shit, man, I can't remember those fractions and stuff."

"Sure you can," I said. "It's all the same from high school. If you review it, it'll all come back to you."

In medical school, I had taught an SAT prep course on the weekends to help pay my living expenses. For kids in more affluent neighborhoods, these courses were standard. But it didn't seem fair, because for Nemesio, his health depended on it.

"Listen," I said. "I'll make you a deal. You go out and buy one of those SAT review books and bring it to our next appointment. I bet we can brush you up on those fractions."

He shifted in his seat and I could just detect a hint of a swagger in his torso. "Okay, Doc. I'll take you on."

Nemesio stood up to go and then turned quickly back to me. "College ain't so bad, but what I really want is to play basketball."

Now it was my turn to nod. "There's nothing like a good ballgame. I played point guard in college."

"You? You even shorter than me."

"That's why I had to find another career."

He grinned. "You and me both." Nemesio put his ski hat on and pulled it carefully down over his forehead. Then he slouched out the door.

———✺———

Nemesio and I met three times over the next two months. While my stethoscope and blood pressure cuff sat idle, we reviewed algebra, analogies, geometry, and reading comprehension. With only a little prodding, Nemesio was able to recall what he had learned in high school. And he thought it was "really cool" when I showed him the tricks and shortcuts that I knew from the SAT prep course.

I lost touch with Nemesio after that. Many days I thought about him, wondering how things turned out. If this were a movie, he'd score a perfect 1600 and be off to Princeton on full scholarship. But Harlem isn't Hollywood, and the challenges in real life are infinitely more complex. I don't know if Nemesio ever got into college—any college—or if he even took the SAT exam. But he did learn a bit more about fractions, and I learned a bit more about the meaning of preventative medicine. At the end of each visit, I would face the clinic billing sheet. The top fifty diagnoses were listed—the most common and important medical issues, according to Medicaid, that our patients faced. I scrutinized them each time, because I was required to check one off, to check off Nemesio Rios's most salient medical diagnosis and treatment, to identify the most pressing issues for his health, to categorize the medical interventions deemed necessary for this patient's well-being; otherwise the clinic wouldn't get reimbursed.

SAT prep was not among them.

CHAPTER ELEVEN

TENDRILS

"DOCTORA?" A KNOCK ON MY OFFICE DOOR. "I no have appointment, but maybe you can tell me results of *la biopsia?*" An edgy scent of ripe flowers enters with her.

Have I seen this woman in my office before? She looks vaguely familiar—reddish-blond hair from a bottle, neatly buttoned polyester blouse just one half-step away from mainstream American style, heavy-lidded brown eyes. But half of my practice is middle-aged Hispanic women and I can't place her. I certainly can't remember her name. "May I see your clinic card, please?" I ask, relying on my best trick in these situations. She hands me the plastic red card with embossed letters like print for the blind that every Bellevue patient carries. *Concepcion Mendoza, 1372714.*

I type her number into the computer and I see that a biopsy was performed three days ago but no results are back yet. It isn't even clear from the computer what part of the body has been biopsied. I haven't ordered a biopsy on any of my patients in the recent past, yet this woman feels familiar. The floral humidity that enters with her is claiming my small office. I imagine she is recreating her tropical homeland here in the concrete jungle of New York on this dark winter day. Is she one of my patients?

Obviously yes, if she knows who I am and is coming to me for results. I can't admit to her that I don't remember. There are just too many patients.

"Not yet, *señora*. Maybe in a few days." I try to make it sound like I know about the biopsy.

"Ah, *sí, Doctora.*"

"I'll call you when the results are back."

"*Sí, Doctora. Gracias.*" She makes a small bow as she backs out with her sultry perfume. Is it jasmine? Maybe hibiscus?

I whisk out the notebook in which I keep copies of my clinic notes—handy when the patient arrives for an appointment but the chart is wandering elsewhere in the bowels of Bellevue. Mendoza, Mendoza. I leaf through the pink pages. Yes, here it is. Concepcion Mendoza. Two months ago, in late October, she was here for her first visit. Now I am starting to remember.

> **CHIEF COMPLAINT:** 68-year-old Argentinean woman with no past medical history comes to clinic complaining of "cyst" under right arm.

Every patient's history starts the same way, with the dangle of a vine that just grazes your cheek. Once the threshold of the chief complaint is crossed—once a hand has reached instinctively toward the tendril skimming the cheek—the doctor has now plunged into the thicket of the patient's history. It was these histories that began to pile up within me. Each with their beckoning chief complaints. Carola Castaña with her swollen hands. Lester Karlin with pain both outside and in. Wilbur Reston with his overarching depression. The young Navajo woman with acne. Each of their chief complaints blossomed into full lives that lured me into their complexities, enveloped me in their nuances. As I took these patients' histories, they grew around me, within me, and I within them.

> **CC:** 68-year-old Argentinean woman with no past medical history comes to clinic complaining of "cyst" under right arm.

Ah, yes. I remember now. I remember that visit clearly now: the heavy-lidded eyes, the floral edginess, the weighted guttural consonants of her Argentinean Spanish. These fragments coalesce and

I can now see her sitting in the plastic yellow chair next to my desk explaining her problem.

I glance farther down on the page to the physical exam. *No mass or cyst noted in axilla,* my handwriting says. *No breast mass palpated.* That's right, I hadn't felt anything. I'd pressed and prodded under her arm and then did a full breast exam, but I didn't feel anything out of the ordinary. "*Todo está bien,*" I'd told her. I had reassured her and ordered a routine mammogram since she was due for one anyhow. Just a mammogram. I certainly didn't order a biopsy because there was nothing to biopsy.

Something is fishy here. Who ordered the biopsy? And what exactly was biopsied? I continue reading my note.

> **PAST MEDICAL HISTORY:** none. Family History: mother has diabetes. Medications: none. Allergies: none. No recent PAP or mammogram. Describes overall good health.

A frond slinks around my back—tickling, encircling, tightening. I am slowly being pulled into her history, into her life.

> **SOCIAL HISTORY:** born in Buenos Aires. Moved to NY six years ago. Married, no children. Works in a sweater factory. Husband drives taxi. Doesn't smoke, drink, or use drugs.

Over the years, the histories piled up. They grew heavy and lush, both nourishing and choking me with their copiousness. A profusion of sprouting narratives. Ripe live cells dividing and splitting, propagating and widening their reach from the patient to the parents to the children and eventually to me, as we all are gradually entwined in this ever-expanding web. Marianne Binet's brother and sister-in-law. Nazma Uddin's daughter Azina. Diana Rakower and her boyfriend. Nemesio Rios and his family. The endless intergrowth.

These histories both enriched and burdened me. By the end of medical school and residency training at Bellevue I'd had to escape to the jungle for air. But the histories came with me, circling at my feet. Hiking at 10,000 feet of altitude in Peru, puffing without oxygen, and the histories still trailed me. Even now as an attending I still couldn't escape. Was Wilbur Reston still taking care of his puppy? Did Nemesio Rios ever take the SAT and get into college? Insistent creepers, endlessly seeking to propagate. Did Russell McCreary ever get out of Riker's and finally accept his diabetes? Was Cheryl Holloway still touring hospitals for drugs? The raspy leaves chafed my calves, tugging insistently. How did Mr. Yang do with his cancer? Was Marianne Binet ever able to return home, or did she end up in a permanent nursing home?

The writing started in little bits. A scribbled anecdote here, a character profile there. And they spilled out so easily, these histories, these lives; they'd become my history and my life. My history of becoming a doctor and evolving as a person. I started writing about my patients, but now I'm writing about me. In a jungle, they say, you often can't tell which root system connects to which leaves.

I check the computer a few days later. *Preliminary results of biopsy taken from 5x8 centimeter clinically palpable mass of right axilla.*

The vine suddenly tightens.

Five by eight centimeters? That's the size of an orange!

I snatch my notes and read them again. *No mass or cyst noted in axilla*, my handwriting insists. Could I have missed an orange? That's not possible! There must be some mistake. The coil constricts and ensnares; my breathing feels choked.

The radiologist! The radiologist probably ordered the biopsy. The radiologist must have felt the mass during the mammogram and then sent Mrs. Mendoza for a biopsy. But could I have missed an orange-size mass, or had it grown from the time I'd seen her?

Breast tissue normal on physical exam, the report continues its narrative, *but suspicious axillary mass noted. Preliminary results suggest carcinoma.* The branches have suddenly enveloped the two of us in a strangling grip. Three days ago I'd barely recognized Concepcion Mendoza standing in my doorway, and now our lives and histories have clenched into a chafing knot.

It was only two months ago that she had her first appointment with me. Could that *thing* have grown so much in two months? In the time it took to get a routine mammogram (damn it, Bellevue, why is everything so goddamn slow?) could that *thing* that I couldn't even feel have grown into an orange, into a cancer? The knotted brambles are scratchy and unsettle my body as I try to rearrange it into a comfortable position in the squeaky office chair.

It's still only the preliminary results, I remind myself. That's what the words in the computer say, *preliminary results.* It could still be an error. I have to wait for the final results.

I telephone the lab every day. Concepcion Mendoza is now with me constantly, her heavy floral fragrance trailing me. Any day now, they tell me, trying to reassure me, but I keep calling because the thorns are starting to scratch and draw blood.

⸺⁓⸺

Words fly everywhere in this business. The words of the chief complaint. The words of the diagnosis. Be specific, we attendings tell the students. Choose your words carefully. Don't just say *pneumonia* when you mean "pneumococcal pneumonia of the left lower lobe accompanied by bacteremia."

Words are so easy, sometimes too easy, and too meaningless. Weightless, they tumble effortlessly into the air and onto the page. But they can carry such different weights in different situations.

Pneumonia. Is it the pneumonia of the twenty-five-year-old who will be back playing soccer after a few days of antibiotic pills, the one that will easily be forgotten the next time a doctor asks about his medical history? Or is it the pneumonia of the intubated patient in the ICU with renal failure and end-stage emphysema, the pneumonia that in Osler's terms is "the old man's friend," the one that brings swift, forgiving death?

Words. Words of the histories that I take from my patients.

Words of the biopsy reports. Words of how I explain to patients. Words of the stories that I write down. The branches of the stories grow so tangled that sometimes I can't remember what goes with whom. I can't keep them in the nice ordered narratives of the novels that I love. Lives don't work like fiction. The endings confound, the characters are contradictory, the plots are frustratingly out of my control. I can't create seamless stories with gratifying endings.

What do I say?

⸺ ❧ ⸺

That treacly lemon-yellow paper they use for official reports now sits on my desk. SQUAMOUS CELL CARCINOMA. All capital letters in irritating dot-matrix print. METASTATIC.

I call her all day on Wednesday. She works in the sweater factory and has no answering machine at home. I take her phone number home with me in the evening and try again. No answer.

No answer, thank goodness. What would I say on the telephone?

Thursday. Friday. The weekend is coming. Should I ruin her weekend? But I should tell her as soon as possible. But if I wait until Monday, what difference will two days make?

Monday day. I avoid the phone. Monday night. Okay, I must call. I can't keep putting this off. But what am I going to say? I can't tell her over the phone.

But she'll know something is bad no matter what I say. Why else would I say that I have to see her in my office right away? What if she insists on knowing over the phone? After all, she has a job, and it's hard to get to the clinic.

Tuesday day. The phone haunts me. Tuesday night. I dial her number from my home.

"Hello? *Señora? La doctora aquí. Cómo está?*" Sound casual, like it's no big deal that I'm calling at 9:00 P.M. Just calling to say hi. "Do you think you could come to my office, *mañana?*

"Anytime—before work, after work, no problem.

"No, you don't need an appointment, just tell the clerk that I'm expecting you.

"*La biopsia?* No, the results aren't back yet. But I'll get them for you when you come in.

"Yes, it is warm for December. *Feliz Navidades, señora.*"

Yes, I lied. Sort of. Kind of. What am I supposed to say? Yes, it is warm for December. Yes, it is metastatic. Could have originated from the lung or esophagus or larynx... could be from anywhere. But I'm sure it will snow in time for Christmas.

<hr>

Wednesday morning, 7:30 A.M. The clerks haven't even arrived yet, but I'm waiting in my office. It's an hour before my regularly scheduled patients, but it's the only time she could come and still get to the factory on time.

The *Dictionario Español-Ingles* is primed, waiting at my elbow. Test forms are clenched in my hand: bone scan, CT scan, X-ray, blood tests. I write the oncology referral while I wait in the morning silence. *68-year-old Argentinean woman with no PMH...*

I have this cyst, *Doctora*, under my arm. Some days I feel it, some days I don't.

I don't feel anything, *señora*.

No mass or cyst noted in axilla. No breast mass palpated.

I don't feel anything, *señora*, but we'll get a *mammograma* anyway. You need a regular *mammograma* at your age.

The official pathology report sits on top of the pile in my hand. The yellow paper is nauseating to look at and the all-capital letters refuse to let my eyes or mind wander elsewhere. BREAST TISSUE NORMAL, BUT SUSPICIOUS AXILLARY MASS NOTED. CLINICAL CORRELATION ADVISED.

SUSPICIOUS AXILLARY MASS. What strange words we use in medicine. Suspicious mass. Suspicious of whom? Suspicious of what?

CLINICAL CORRELATION ADVISED, the report suggests. Thank you, great advice. Really helpful.

Correlation?

I have this cyst, *Doctora*.

No mass or cyst noted in axilla. Nothing correlates.

There's a knock on my door. "*Buenos días, señora.*"

"*Buenos días, Doctora.*"

Edgy flowers nervously cast their scent. I smell the humid lushness of South America. I grope for my Spanish.

I love the English language. So many nuances, so many synonyms. An endlessly malleable piece of clay, honed by decades of my nonchalant use. But now I must negotiate with inflexible tools. Back to a grammar-school lexicon.

"*Señora...*" I struggle for words to speak while the ones on the paper scorch my fingers. SQUAMOUS CELL CARCINOMA, METASTATIC. Harsh metallic words.

"*Señora...*" I try again. SQUAMOUS CELL. Latin: flattened, scaly cells. Pancakes stacked delicately like bricks to form a protective wall—firm yet flexible. Mighty bastion surrounding each organ, guarding against enemy attack. But now infiltrated by alien forces.

"*La biopsia está...*" CARCINOMA. Greek: crab. A crab that slinks in the darkness, insinuating its pincers into the sinews of the body, sucking out the marrow.

"*Es grave, Doctora?*"

"*Si, señora, es grave.*" METASTATIC. Greek. *Meta:* over, beyond. *Stasis:* standing. Gone from this standing, venturing beyond this place, seeking nutrient riches, pillaging anything in its path. Arrived in the axilla as an evil emissary from somewhere else. I just don't know from where.

The words manage to crawl between us. "*El tumor...*" "*La quimioterapia.*" Her Argentinean accent challenges me, and I'm sure my pastiche of Mexican–Peruvian–Guatemalan–New Yorkian Spanish makes her squint. But cancer has such a talent for linguistic clarity. Exhausting my supply of conjugable verbs, I reach for a pen. I scribble a phone number on the back of the blood test form and point to my beeper. "*Toda los días. Y los noches.*"

Years of medical training have brought me to this moment. The moment where I can help her negotiate through the complicated workup of metastatic cancer. I know what tests need to be done and what treatments can be offered without having to ask someone else. It has also brought me to the moment where I can begin to help her negotiate through her fears and the unknown. When I embarked upon this voyage as a beginning medical student I knew about gaining the former skills, but I couldn't have comprehended that the latter skills would be so crucial.

I had thought that becoming a doctor would entail learning everything about the human body; I hadn't thought much beyond that. I had no idea that I would have to open myself up to my patients' histories and listen for the unspoken. As the poet John Stone once said to a class of graduating medical students, "You will learn to see most acutely out of the corner of your eye, to hear best with your inner ear." I had no understanding that my patients' histories would create my history.

When I studied for my medical boards I remember being overwhelmed by the amount of knowledge I had to absorb. I was awed and humbled by the sheer vastness and the challenge of mastering it. But now that seems like the easy part. All I had to do for that was keep cramming and memorizing. It's the other challenge, that of stepping into the emotional fray with the patient, that truly awes and humbles me. It is in that unsettling zone in which healing has a chance to take place.

I don't recall the moment when I realized that I'd become a doctor, that I'd actually arrived at that coveted destination. Did it happen when I received my medical diploma? When I completed residency? Was it the first time I ran a successful code? The first time I prescribed a medicine without asking anyone for advice? Or the first time I couldn't fall asleep because I was worrying about a patient? I suppose becoming a doctor is like one of those vines that wends perpetually through the jungle. It draws nourishment from the trees it coils around and the bushes it encounters along its journey, but it is impossible to clearly demarcate its beginning or end.

I walk with Mrs. Mendoza upstairs to the radiology suite—the CT scan needs to be done immediately. I point out where the bone scan room is. That also needs to be done right away. My patients will be arriving in the clinic shortly and I must go now. I hand her the stack of papers for all of the tests, along with an absence note for work, and then we stand still for a moment, contemplating the silent space between us. She reaches her arms forward and we hug. I feel the papers for the CT scan and the bone scan at my back as the softness of her floral perfume surrounds me. The tendrils have enfolded us and our histories have now joined.

POSTSCRIPT

Mrs. Mendoza's tumor turned out to have come from a small skin cancer on her hand that had been removed one year prior—something she'd considered so trivial that she never even thought to mention it as part of her medical history.

She underwent radiation and surgical removal of the tumor in her axilla and returned to work shortly thereafter. We cheered that it had turned out to be just a local cancer and was so easy to treat.

Six months later, as I was writing this essay, she came to my office with a rubbery bump on her shoulder. I sent her for a biopsy immediately, but before the results were even back, she was admitted to a hospital in Brooklyn with a stroke. For a moment I was relieved, thinking that this was just an "ordinary" stroke, from which she might easily recover.

But the doctor called to tell me that there were metastases in the brain and innumerable masses in her lung—the largest being the size of a grapefruit. It was no ordinary stroke; the metastatic journey continued unabated.

There was no phone in Mrs. Mendoza's room, so I couldn't call her; in any case, she couldn't speak. I made plans to go visit her that Saturday, but her sister called me on Friday night to say she'd passed away. Sad that I had been unable to see her when she was alive, I attended her viewing in a tiny funeral home in the Sunset Park section of Brooklyn. Five people—her sister, her husband, and three friends from the Argentinean community—were there. I added my flowers to the heaping pile on her open coffin. The lush, tropical scent caught in my throat. I said good-bye.

CHAPTER TWELVE

MISSING THE FINAL ACT

DISEASES, LIKE DRAMAS, HAVE NATURAL progressions: introductions, backgrounds, developments, climaxes, and denouements. And each disease of each person has its own singular tempo. Often the natural rhythms are unpredictable, with sudden overnight developments or stultifyingly dull periods of waiting. Life in a teaching hospital, however, is paced by the hard-edged specifics of the academic calendar. When I attend on the medical wards, I do so for exactly four weeks at a time. After twenty-eight days of intense involvement in my patients' lives, I must abandon the ward to return to my home base in the clinic—irrespective of the progression of their individual dramas.

Today is the twenty-eighth day of my month on the wards. A quiet Sunday morning of rounds. I arrive early, even before the interns, because there are so many patients to see. There is, of course, the absurdity of seeing the newly admitted patients today, of introducing myself as the attending physician at the same time as I say that this is my last day and that they will meet new doctors tomorrow. But it has to be done.

And then there are the patients who have been here for a few days or even a few weeks. These are the patients whom I've come to know, whose dramas I've witnessed in the making but whose final acts I will miss. It all seems so bizarre. Aren't doctors supposed to stay with their patients until the bitter end?

Most patients, however, are understanding. They've been in the academic system before and have grown accustomed to—or at least tolerant of—hordes of medical students, interns, residents, fellows, and attendings parading in and out of their rooms. Most don't know the distinction between these varying levels of the medical hierarchy, and most, frankly, don't seem to care. The medical student's unhurried afternoons of conversation probably mean more to a patient than the fact that the attending physician is board-certified in her medical specialty.

Rishala, a sweet-faced twenty-three-year-old, is stuck in the hospital for six weeks of intravenous antibiotics for an abdominal abscess. Our lives crossed during her weeks two through five. I have seen only a bouncy Indian woman eager and impatient to return to her studies as a respiratory therapist. She seems too healthy to be here, but I have read in her chart what week one was like, when she was prostrate with a fever of 105 degrees, consumed by abdominal pain, too weak even to walk. I missed the endless X-rays and CT scans and blood cultures and the various misdiagnoses of pancreatitis and gallstones.

I waltzed on to the scene during Act II, when the broad-spectrum antibiotics had already restored her energy and appetite. Now she is achingly bored with confinement and my visits have been mainly to cheer her up rather than alter her medical care. When I told her of a previous patient of mine who studied Italian during his hospital stay, Rishala giggled and whispered that she'd always wanted to learn Spanish. I brought her one of my basic Spanish books and each day thereafter she has greeted me with "*Cómo está?*" and her new vocabulary word of the day. Now I am leaving the week before her antibiotic course is complete. We've had a month of daily chats about movies, abscesses, and Spanish conjugations, but I will not be able to partake in the climax and denouement of her drama. I will not be able to celebrate the sweetness of her discharge or her mastery of the past participle.

Anjali is another Indian woman on my service. She is only forty-five, but the furrows etched around her eyes speak of other forces aging her. Twenty years ago she had a routine gallbladder operation in India and the doctors recommended a blood transfusion because she seemed a bit weak at the edges. Along with the oxygen-rich red blood cells, the hepatitis C virus was transfused into her veins, and decades later her liver began to fail.

Now she is near the end stages, with intractable fluid swelling her petite body. This time the fluid is infected, and she, like Rishala, requires six weeks of intravenous antibiotics. Her only hope would be a liver transplant. She is a perfect candidate: never drank alcohol, never used drugs, young, reliable, no other medical problems, has a supportive family. Except for one thing: she isn't an American citizen.

Anjali cried frequently during the month and it was often excruciatingly uncomfortable to remain in her room. Every day that I saw her we spoke sadly about the situation; it was impossible to make small talk about the weather. She was an excellent cook, her sons told me. I brought in an Indian cookbook I'd purchased long ago but never used. Anjali spent her days examining the recipes and highlighting the ones she thought were tasty and sufficiently uncomplicated for a busy doctor. I'm leaving before her antibiotics are finished. I am saying good-bye midway through her drama, and she cries when she returns the cookbook to me. She stayed up late last night getting through the final chapter on desserts. After this month the cookbook will sit untouched on my shelf. I will remain sadly ignorant of the final chapter of her story and it will be too painful to prepare those recipes.

Karolina was admitted to our service not even forty-eight hours ago. I barely know her and now I am saying good-bye. She is twenty-one; our medical service seems particularly young this month. A frail wisp of a young woman who speaks little English, she nods as I try to say both hello and good-bye in the same breath. When she was vomiting every day in her native Poland, she was diagnosed with anorexia and bulimia. An endoscopy of her stomach had been performed, but apparently no biopsies were taken and nothing seemed amiss. When she arrived in America, she was promptly admitted to the psychiatric ward for severe anorexia. Another endoscopy was performed, however, and gastric cancer was there, clear as summer, and already Stage IV—metastatic. I feel guilty leaving so early in the game with Karolina. There will be long and serious talks in the next few weeks, but I am bailing out. Though at least she speaks enough English to say good-bye.

Xi-Lang doesn't speak a single word of English. Not one. She is forty-one and has Stage IV metastatic cervical cancer. She's been in the hospital for a week and has already signed a DNR. Planning for hospice care is well under way. Since I can't normally locate the Cantonese interpreter for my daily rounds, I simply smile at her and hope my eyes convey my concern. "*Tong?*" I ask, using the only word in Chinese that I know. "Pain? *Tong?*" I ask again, pointing to her belly. She shakes her head no; her morphine is adequate. Her husband comes every evening with their two young children. It is simply too agonizing to watch, especially without being able to communicate, and often I find myself backing quickly out the door. I tell myself that it's because we have nothing to say, but I know it is otherwise. On this Sunday I say good-bye in the most basic of ways. I take her hand in mine and shake it slowly. Then I smile and wave good-bye like a small child would—cheerily and probably too demonstratively. In the absence of words my gestures feel overly dramatic and I am acutely aware of their awkwardness. I point from my heart to hers and I think she understands.

I have finished seeing all my patients and am jotting the last of the progress notes in their charts. My twenty-eight days are drawing to a close. What a month it has been. So many young people, it seems, this month. So many young women. All with such horrible illnesses. It's not always like this, and of course there were many patients—men and women—who were in and out in a matter of days as their asthma attacks or pneumonias easily resolved. But it's the ones with cancer and serious infections who stay for long periods of time. My canvas of time and their canvas of time will overlap only partially. For some patients, like Karolina, the overlap will be their Act I. For others, like Anjali, it will be their

Act III. And there were those this month for whom I bore witness to their final act.

Why does this leave me so unsettled? It is, of course, impossible for me to be here round-the-clock, every day, every month, for every patient. I have to say good-bye at some point. Three separate months per year of full-time inpatient medicine is all I can handle. It is exhausting in a way that outpatient medicine in the clinic can never be. I do enjoy the opportunity of brushing up on my inpatient skills and there is an excitement to caring for critically ill patients. But the disjointedness imposed by the calendar gnaws under my skin like a persistent parasite.

In the clinic I have the opportunity to live in parallel with my patients, to meet their children and grandchildren, to celebrate their retirements, to mourn the deaths of their parents or spouse. I have been with some of my patients for more than a decade. But whenever I attend on the inpatient wards, a shadow of guilt trails behind me with silent but insistent footsteps. I can never be there enough. I can never be there for the whole story for every patient.

Perhaps this is the deal we must make with our patients in academic medicine. We doctors provide high-level medical care, but at the end of twenty-eight days I exit abruptly, like the annoying theater patron who squeezes out of her row in the middle of the performance, stumbling over purses and knees and programs, apologizing in a hurried whisper. The other audience members shake their heads in the wake of her awkward departure and wonder how she could possibly be so oblivious to the riveting drama upon the stage.

CHAPTER THIRTEEN

EMIGRATION

IN 1915 MY GRANDFATHER IRVING, then age seventeen, stood on a London pier with a one-way steamer ticket clutched in his hand. His mother and seven siblings had already made it this far from Latvia. Their father had stayed, unable to rally behind his wife's convictions that life in the shtetl could only get worse and that it was worth abandoning all that they possessed to set forth into an unknown world. Now Irving and one brother would be the first emissaries to America, to experiment in this strange place and then shepherd the rest of the family from London, one by one.

I try to imagine how it must have felt as he boarded the ship that would take him to this unknown land of America. There was the long and unpleasant journey first, replete with physical discomforts and ample seasickness. And then there would be the arrival at this place, this America that everyone talked so much about. This America that he had been promised would be a land of wealth and opportunity, a magical place that had no equal, something so special that it was worth gambling everything for. At this moment, gazing at the steamship, he would have no words or images to create America in his mind. He would likely have everyone else's opinions and promises of riches, but he himself would possess no vocabulary with which to articulate any internal vision. And of course, he literally did not possess the language of English. He would simply have to take it on faith that this journey, this plunge into the unknown without the ability to turn back, would be worthwhile.

Here I sit, more than ninety years later, with a similar feeling inside. I am halfway through my first pregnancy and have just seen our baby's image up on the ultrasound screen this morning. Suddenly it is so real. I feel like I am traveling to a strange land, one that everyone promises is filled with riches and reward and will be worth all the sacrifices. I possess no vocabulary to articulate the vision and indeed I do not speak the language. I can only rely on everyone else's assurances of how worthwhile it will be. And of course, there is no turning back; it is a one-way ticket.

There is even a similar journey to get there, one of many months and involving a significant amount of nausea. Although the circumstances are different, I'd like to think that I am sharing with my grandfather the awe and fear of the one-way trip to a strange and mysterious land. I see a split-screen image with each of us landing on a crowded dock, squinting in the piercing sunlight, exhausted from the journey, bewildered at the chaos, with no vocabulary and no map, nervous but excited. With no choice but to go forward, we place one tentative foot in front of the other and totter ahead, relying on our inner strengths and instincts to spontaneously invent this new life.

Frankly, I know that my journey takes a whole lot less courage than my grandfather's did. And both pale beside the courage of my great-grandmother Ida, who took the first step, bundling up her eight children and abandoning the only home she'd known, willing to give up everything, including her obstinate husband, to set out for a Promised Land.

I never met Ida, but I have heard many stories about her from my family. Sitting here in the New World, not more than two miles from Ellis Island, where she and her children arrived, I suddenly feel so connected. Through my biological journey, I just might have a touch of insight into what they were feeling.

I, too, am convinced (mostly) that the journey will be worthwhile, that the disorientation upon arrival will eventually dissipate, that I will eventually stop looking and sounding like a greenhorn, that I will soon speak the language fluently and someday be able to casually give advice to others considering the journey. This is what keeps me going—and, of course, the knowledge that there's no turning back. The fact that Irving and Ida succeeded gives me hope that I will also.

Last week my in-laws took us to the Lower East Side to buy silver candlesticks. Grand Street Silver has changed little since Irving and Ida lived in this neighborhood. The owners are Eastern European refugees from the Holocaust, with thick Yiddish accents. As we hunt through the dusty shelves crammed with all manner of Kiddush cups, menorahs, and candlesticks, the news that we are expecting a baby percolates out. The owners are genuinely excited, showering us with *mazel tovs*, knowing that the candlesticks we buy from them will be enjoyed by our child and perhaps passed along as family heirlooms. My grandfather can't be with us to share in our happiness, but this European couple feels like a link to him.

Candlesticks in tow, we trundle through the neighborhood, stopping at Moishe's kosher bakery for rye bread and Gus's sidewalk pickle stand for a quart of half-sours. Most stores in the area now sport signs in Chinese or Spanish, but there are a few still in Yiddish. My grandfather's footprints are still here. His journey brought me here. As a child, I shared with him the love of sculpting and of spinning corny puns. As I nibble on the plain rye bread to keep down the heartburn and queasiness of *my* journey, I smile to myself that we are sharing yet again.

When I prepared to give birth to my first baby, I debated about whether or not to give birth at my own hospital. It wasn't that I was so concerned about anonymity, but there is something odd about being a patient in your own hospital. But it's also known that our hospital takes good care of its own.

Bellevue had just built several beautiful birthing rooms, complete with hot tubs, chintz curtains, cushioned rocking chairs, and queen-size beds for the mother and her partner to stay overnight. These rooms were only for the patients of the midwives—and

I had no opposition to giving birth with a midwife, but if you wanted an epidural, you had to exit these idyllic surroundings and head over to the regular labor floor. The labor floor was undergoing renovations and had a stronger resemblance to a construction zone than a Victorian boudoir.

Up the block at NYU there were also birthing rooms, but they were not nearly as homey and lacked both the hot tub and the overnight bed (after delivery you'd have to relocate to the postpartum unit). But you could get an epidural in your birthing room.

In the end, as it happens for so many of my patients, it was my health insurance plan that decided; NYU—not Bellevue—was the hospital on their plan, and that was that. As a faculty member of the department of medicine at NYU, though one who worked exclusively at Bellevue, NYU could still be considered home. I assumed there would be relative anonymity on the department of obstetrics ward at NYU since I never spent time there and the nurses didn't know me. Before I entered the hospital, I promised myself that I wouldn't pull rank, that I wouldn't use my faculty position to gain any extra privileges, that I would just be a regular patient.

When my contractions became unbearable, my husband and I walked over to NYU. Hoping to avoid crowds, I steered him toward the employee elevators near the cafeteria. But I hadn't realized how un-anonymous a nine-months'-pregnant woman grasping a pillow is, and two security guards materialized with a wheelchair before I could even push the Up button.

"I'm not sick," I started to say, recoiling from that ultimate symbol of dependency. But another contraction slugged me and I sank gratefully into the chair.

I was wheeled into the OB ward, my faculty ID card on its necklace jostling over my belly. Once placed in a room, I was handed one of those dreadful blue patient gowns, and I thought, This is it. This is the low point. The gown was every bit as horrible as I imagined it would be when I saw it on my patients. It was uncomfortable, the ties on the neck were too loose, causing it to sag, and the ties on the back weren't in the right places, making every step an opportunity to expose oneself to the general public.

In walked the anesthesia resident to place the epidural. He was a pleasant young fellow, and he began to explain the procedure. I cut him short. "No offense intended," I said politely, "but please send in your attending."

"But I'm a third-year resident; I've put in hundreds of these," he said, the umbrage palpable in his expression.

I smiled my kindest, most educational smile—after all, I was still an attending physician and every moment was still a teaching moment. "I have all the respect in the world for residents, but not when I'm having contractions you can measure on the Richter scale. Now, please page your attending."

He grimaced and then sighed. I agreed to let him put in the IV but not before I negotiated location and needle size; I managed to bargain him down one gauge smaller. We both winced—for different reasons—when the IV did not go in on the first try.

The anesthesia attending arrived and put in the epidural. I hollered when the lidocaine was injected, knowing full well that I'd always blithely assured my patients that it would be "just a little burning" whenever I injected lidocaine. It was more like a hot poker rooting around in my back, slicing into my muscles and bones.

The nurse bustled about, affixing the fetal monitor to my belly. The machine next to me sprang to life, with buttons, dials, and screens glittering. Skinny strips of black scribbles began slithering out of the machine, piling up on the floor like a knot of snakes. It resembled an EKG machine gone wild. I watched the data—*my* data—crumple onto the floor, with a mix of discomfort and confusion. Occasionally, the nurse or the obstetrician would grab a handful of moving paper, stare at it with furrowed brow, then tear a segment off, leaving the rest to accumulate as detritus on the floor.

My intellect overcame my sense of disembodiedness, and I

commenced a lecture aimed at the nurse about how unnecessary testing in healthy patients leads to more false positives than true positives, thus exposing more populations to adverse outcomes. She just smiled benignly...then another contraction ripped through me.

The contractions and the fetal heart rate weren't coinciding to the satisfaction of my obstetrician, and so he called in one of the house staff to assist with fetal scalp monitoring. In walked an intern I recognized from Bellevue. She smiled politely, if a bit awkwardly, at me. I could only groan. They say that a pregnant woman is ready to deliver when privacy issues cease to register, and for all she cares it could be the postman down there between her legs.

Through my haze of pain, nausea, and humiliation, I could sense that a teaching moment was occurring down there. The obstetrician—the attending—was guiding the intern through a scalp pH procedure. They were drawing a tiny bit of blood from my baby's scalp to check the acidity level. This would be the most accurate measure of whether the baby was getting enough oxygen during my contractions. I could hear the intern and attending muttering between themselves as they performed the procedure. I felt a ping of altruism for my contribution to the medical education process, but hoped against hope—both for the intern and for me—that the intern's inexperience wouldn't necessitate a repeat procedure.

The obstetrician announced that he wasn't happy with the pH, and the nurse immediately slapped an oxygen mask on my face. A reflex in me insisted on retaining medical control over the situation; if there was a pH value floating around, I wanted to know precisely how acidotic my baby's blood was. I demanded to know what the pH reading was, or at least I attempted to demand. It was suddenly such an effort to form the words and to move the muscles of my parched mouth, and the oxygen mask muffled my efforts to make myself heard.

On my third request, the pH was finally reported to me. The number floated into my ears and wobbled toward my consciousness, jiggling helplessly between synapses, seemingly unable to glue itself to a neuron. I struggled to retain it in my memory, but I could feel it slipping helplessly out of my awareness. I closed my eyes and let my head fall back on the pillow, hoping the obstetrician possessed a sufficient grasp of acid-base physiology.

The intern smiled up at me. "Your baby has a full head of hair," she said. "I had to give it a little haircut in order to get the scalp blood sample. An in-utero haircut." She giggled.

I recognized that as humor that was supposed to relax a patient, but I was too cranky. They drew a second scalp pH and the number was apparently a bit better, but now I had a slight fever, so they started IV antibiotics.

Someone plunked an ice chip in my mouth, and I sucked it gratefully. One of the barbaric features of modern obstetrics is that you are not permitted to eat or drink until a baby has been produced (I think they use food and water as the incentive).

The obstetrician and intern drew a third blood sample from my poor baby's scalp. They sent two tests for pH from the same sample, but the numbers came back different—one good and one bad—and they didn't know which one to believe. The obstetrician and intern began to debate whether the scalp pH readings made any sense at all and whether it was time to start thinking about forceps or let the delivery proceed as it was going.

This indecision somehow crystallized my consciousness for a brief moment. I tore my oxygen mask off. "Don't you guys know anything about evidence-based medicine? The two discordant pH values demonstrate the limits of the operating characteristics of the test. You shouldn't be sending tests if the results won't cause a change in your clinical management. Think before you test!"

The obstetrician didn't seem amused. "OK," he barked, "start pushing. If this baby isn't out in thirty minutes, we're doing a C-section."

⸺⸙⸺

Twenty-nine minutes later, a wrinkly, gooey, splotchy, but indescribably beautiful baby girl emerged. From that moment, everything else simply evaporated.

The cleaning-up and sewing-up postdelivery seemed to take hours. Which was okay with me, as my husband and I were content to be mesmerized by the seven pounds of infant in our arms. But the honeymoon with our baby had to come to an end, and I was once again loaded into the wheelchair (for which I was ever grateful), a precious bundle was placed on my lap, and all my earthly possessions in plastic bags were strung off the back. The whole circus was wheeled into the postpartum unit. My daughter was whisked off to the newborn nursery to face her very first battery of standardized tests. My husband was sent off to Admitting to take care of paperwork.

A nurse eased me into the bed. With a briskly pleasant voice she plopped a frosty pitcher of ice water on my table. "We'll just leave this for you right here." A matching plastic yellow cup sat at its side.

And suddenly, I was alone. Well, not quite alone. Behind the curtain was another woman who'd also just delivered a baby. Neither of us could move much, so we just exchanged exhausted, anonymous hellos.

My first sensation, upon finally leaning back into the bed, was ferocious thirst. The hours of water deprivation suddenly caved in on me with a powerful awareness.

Unfortunately, my beautiful pitcher of ice water had been placed just out of my arm's reach.

Anyone who's been through labor, delivery, and episiotomies, knows that it is not such an easy task to move oneself, even just "right here" or "right there." I attempted various contortions of my arms and upper body, but my fingers fell short of the glistening pitcher. I tried to use my pillow to lasso the liquid, but it was too floppy. Finally I pressed the call button and asked that my water be moved closer.

I shouldn't have been surprised that no one came immediately. I work in a busy city hospital, and I hear all those calls to the nurses' station. "Please move my water" is not very high up on the triage list. Chest pains and difficulty breathing get first priority.

But for me, parched, in pain, and essentially helpless, it was the only thing I could think about. Water, water, water... the words floated on my brain. The droplets that were evaporating tantalizingly on the outside of the plastic pitcher simply served to drive me into dehydrational delirium.

No one came.

I didn't want to be an annoying patient (as a doctor, I'd always hated those), and I knew the nurses were short-staffed and had lots of responsibilities. I tried to be patient, and then I finally buzzed again. "We're changing shift now," came the reply. "Someone will be in shortly."

I grimaced. I knew how important it was for the nurses to converse as they were preparing to hand over care, but I was thirsty, damn it, and I couldn't reach my water.

I remembered how I felt when I did my rounds at Bellevue, my mind working overtime to keep track of the specifics of thirty-five patients' medical care and the teaching of two residents, four interns, and six medical students. I'd be walking fast, talking fast, and cogitating even faster to keep everything successfully juggled. And then a patient would ask for a tissue, or a ginger ale, or a pillowcase. There would be a distinct pinch of annoyance in my head; not that I didn't want to help the patient, but I had hundreds of details swirling in my mind and this little request might disrupt the agonizingly achieved balance.

Couldn't they just wait for the nurse? I wanted to say. I'm too busy with so many very important things. That small request was tiny in significance compared to the weighty matters that I was juggling. Didn't they realize that?

But now I wanted one of those tiny requests. It was more important, at that moment, than any other aspect of my medical care, any aspect of the running of the postpartum unit, of the entire hospital for that matter. It was critical to the survival of the universe as we knew it.

I realized that I had just completed Being a Patient 101, something that decades of medical training and clinical practice had never taught me.

When a nurse aide finally arrived and slid the pitcher the eight inches necessary for it to reach my desperate grip, I felt a swooning relief, a joy like that I've felt when I've done successful CPR on a patient and revived him from the dead.

～∞∞∞～

Several hours later, I marshaled my strength to attempt the three-foot walk to the bathroom. I was desperate to wash up as best I could (another inhumanity of modern obstetrics is that a shower is not permitted in the first twenty-four hours). Anyone who has attended the birth of a baby knows that while it is a perfectly natural process, it is an inordinately messy one.

I limped the few steps to the bathroom, using one hand to bolster my rickety balance and the other to keep that infernal patient gown at least semirespectably closed. Once in the tiny bathroom, I had to devise some creative strategies to wash myself using the sink, the microscopic sliver of soap, the little plastic spray bottle the nurse had given me, and a small pile of paper towels. Under ordinary circumstances, this could be challenging, but now, when it was excruciating to sit, stand, bend, or walk, it was a comedy of the absurd. Water splattered on the floor as I tried to wash the various sections of my body, but I couldn't reach down to wipe up the slippery floor. Mopping with a paper towel under my foot only served to accumulate mushy, wet brown paper towels, which I couldn't possibly bend to pick up. My gown was full of blood and guck, and it had long since slipped to the floor along with reams of other unnameable body fluids.

I strove to delineate a clean/dry zone from a wet/dirty zone, but the latter kept expanding, so I was continually hobbling into an ever-smaller safe zone. My greatest fear was that I would slip and land in the middle of all my accumulated debris and not be able to get up (and not be able to reach the call button that was some-where in the bathroom).

By the time I had finished, I was somewhat cleaner than I'd been, but I had made, literally, a bloody mess of the bathroom. If this hadn't been the postpartum unit, one might have been for-given for thinking it was a crime scene.

Normally a fairly obsessively neat person, my instinct was to plop immediately down on my hands and knees and clean up the mess I had made. But I could barely walk the three steps back to bed.

Immediately I called the nurses' station and explained, apolo-getically, that I'd made a mess of my bathroom and could they please send housekeeping, as I was unable to clean it up myself.

"Someone will be there soon," I was informed.

I eased myself back in my bed, snuggling up with the ice packs —a postpartum woman's best friend. An hour went by, and no one had come to clean the bathroom. I called again, embarrassed that my roommate, or one of her guests, might need to use the bathroom.

"Someone will be there shortly," came the reply.

I tried to make myself comfortable—an absurdly hopeless en-deavor, I learned. Another hour went by, still no action. I called again to complain.

"Someone will be there shortly," came the reply.

I sat in my bed trying to relax but found myself tormented by the thought of all sorts of my body fluids and inner guck strewn about the bathroom. For anyone who is normally fastidious about such things, it is horribly embarrassing.

I called again. No action.

Finally, after what seemed like days but which was probably just a few hours, I called the nurses' station one last time. "This is Dr. Ofri," I barked. "I am an attending physician on faculty here, and the bathroom in my room is a disgusting mess."

Within minutes, a housekeeper materialized, and the bathroom was scrubbed to its original polish and gleam.

Shortly thereafter, my daughter was delivered to me from the nursery, apparently having passed all her tests with flying colors. I spent the rest of the night in both joy and anguish, trying to figure out just how this miracle had managed to spring up in my little world.

———⟨∞⟩———

Being a patient encompasses many things, but I had no idea how much shame and humiliation are a part of the experience: from the horrid gowns that never cover enough, to the exposure of some of the most private and embarrassing bodily functions, to the smells and sights which one is forced to wallow in, to the helplessness and inability to assert one's control.

I knew that I was lucky to have been able to pull strings to get my bathroom cleaned, but most patients can't. I felt guilty that I was able to resort to that and angry that I was forced to.

I know that a brief hospitalization to have a baby doesn't come close to the agony of prolonged illness. Even so, my eyes were opened in a way that years of medical training had not done. We always talk with our students and interns about the need to maintain a patient's dignity, and it seems like such an obvious thing. But until I had the chance to experience an aspect of that (even though it probably ranked on the minor end of the scale of patient indignities) I hadn't really known what that meant.

As doctors, we try to give our patients the best medical care. And when we discuss our patients on rounds, or in our heads, and we've addressed their cardiovascular system, their respiratory system, and their antibiotics, we feel satisfied that we've taken care of all the major issues. But so much more affects the patient's experience. These are minor things in the eyes of the doctor (and in some sense they are indeed minor compared to the critical business of saving lives and preventing major medical complications), but they can feel like life or death for the patient.

Now, when I lead my team on rounds in the hospital, I demonstrate the history-taking and physical-exam skills that I, as the attending physician, wish my interns and students to learn. And then I pull the patient's tray table close to the bed. I assemble the water, the telephone, the tissues, and the call button, so that all are within reach. Occasionally I detect a grumble or an annoyed shifting of body posture from the house staff as precious time is "wasted" with my redecorating endeavors.

But I calmly ignore these and continue my arrangements until everything is in place. I learned a valuable lesson in my brief time as a patient: what matters to patients is not *just* that they are receiving superb medical care, but also that they know they are being cared for, that their human needs are recognized, even if that need is just having a glass of water within reach.

My grandfather eventually became a full-fledged American. By the time I knew him, the customs of American life had completely replaced his greenhorn ways. No one could ever imagine him lost, without language, without a network of connections, without a sense of his life here in this country. But I know that the experience of his emigration never left him; it was a permanent part of his subconscious, and, I think, contributed to his extraordinary sense of compassion for the small things in life.

And I eventually became a full-fledged parent of two. Within a short time, I, too, shed my greenhorn ways and could fully navigate in this new world. I could even offer advice to others who hadn't yet made this trip. And while the immediate sensations of pain during the deliveries has faded, the sensation of being helpless and out of control has not. It is a sensual memory of a unique type that pops up periodically when I make rounds on my own patients, and when I gaze at my own two children, who, at this stage of their lives, are still so utterly dependent upon me.

And while it is always gratifying to arrive at one's destination, it is sometimes during the process of getting there that the most significant and humbling lessons are acquired.

CHAPTER FOURTEEN

TOOLS OF THE TRADE

THE LIST OF PATIENTS WAS CRISP IN MY HAND. Crisp, clear, and un-muddied, as it always is the first day of a new month on the wards. After three months of respite in the clinic, I was once again back on the wards. I knew that the sheet of paper would soon be crumpled and covered with scrawls, as I scurried about meeting thirty-six patients, two residents, four interns, and six medical students. But for now the paper felt cool, controlled, and reliable in my grip.

I was ashamed to admit it, but I was perversely thankful for the numerous comatose patients on my service because they made rounds faster and left more time to concentrate on the active GI bleeders, the patients in diabetic ketoacidosis, the ones with gram-negative septicemia, and the ones who spoke English.

Mrs. Millstein was one such comatose patient, an elderly woman with Alzheimer's disease who'd been sent from her nursing home in Brooklyn after falling and hitting her head. Overflowing hospital census and pure bad luck conspired to land Mrs. Millstein on 7-East, galaxies away, for all practical purposes, from the medical wards on the sixteenth and seventeenth floors. The combination of her flatline mental status and her location in the hinterlands of the hospital ensured that my visits would be brief and infrequent.

The previous attending had told me that he'd spoken with the patient's sister in Florida, the social worker from the nursing home, as well as the patient's rabbi. All assured him that Mrs. Millstein would not want any aggressive measures. A DNR had been signed and the plan was to place a permanent feeding tube then return the patient to her nursing home.

I poked my head in Mrs. Millstein's room on that first day on the wards. I saw a white-haired elderly lady, either sleeping or unconscious, but clearly comfortable. She was breathing well and her vitals were stable. I nodded to myself, checked off the box on my now slightly rumpled list of patients, and continued with my rounds.

I had no plans to call the sister—or do any additional work for this patient—since the previous attending had settled the main issues, and a clearly defined plan was in place. But then the question arose as to whether Mrs. Millstein would have considered the planned permanent feeding tube to be invasive, and this decision would require consultation with the family. So I dialed the phone number and a heavily Eastern European–accented voice met my ears. "Yes, I am Goldie. I am her sister."

I explained to Goldie that I was taking care of her sister, that I was the new doctor on the wards. She told me that Dora would never want any painful or invasive procedures. We agreed that a permanent feeding tube would not be necessary, that the temporary tube was okay, given Mrs. Millstein's comatose state and likely abbreviated life expectancy, and that the patient would not get any IVs or blood draws. "Dora was a very cheerful person," Goldie told me. "Everybody loved her."

I paused, looking up from the furrowed and rutted patient list on which I'd been jotting the notes of our conversation. Cheerful, I mused, turning my hands over. It was always hard to imagine a comatose patient ever having been cheerful.

The transfer process moved along. Papers were signed and stamped. Transportation services were arranged. Necessary authorizations were obtained. On the day of transfer, as I readied myself to cross one more patient off my now well-worn list, the social worker noted the last set of vital signs. There was a fever.

The great machinations of interhospital transfer ground to a halt: nobody, it seemed, could be transferred anywhere, anytime, at any stage of illness, with a core body temperature other than 98.6 degrees. Despite my protestations that the patient was already receiving oral antibiotics, that she would not undergo blood cultures or be given IV antibiotics, that she had a DNR order, that the medical team would not do anything about this fever, that in fact it was actually *expected* that this patient would have a fever, the social work rule was ironclad. I would not be able to cross Mrs. Millstein off my list.

It was already quite late in the day, but I decided to call to Goldie. I assumed we could have a quick conversation and that she would be in agreement with my judgment that her sister could indeed return to her nursing home despite the peregrinations of her body temperature. I glanced at my watch as I dialed her number, packing my stethoscope and crumpled patient list in my bag to leave for the evening. Goldie sounded delighted to hear from me. She asked me if Dora looked comfortable, and I said yes.

"Dora had such a hard life," Goldie said. "I am much younger and she was like a mother to me." In the casual voice of someone recounting her afternoon shopping, she added, "We went through the camps together, you know. She took care of me after we lost our parents. She is the reason I survived."

My hands abruptly ceased their activity and drew together with interlocked fingers, awkwardly making their way down into my lap. Goldie and I proceeded to talk for the better part of an hour. Goldie told me about Dora's escape in Europe, their harrowing adventures in the forest, their long journey to America.

After the phone call, I went back to Mrs. Millstein's room. I put down my bag, pulled up the empty visitors' chair, and sat next to Mrs. Millstein. Next to Dora. The sun had already set over the East River, and the darkness from the windows was a rigid wall of black behind me. I looked at Dora under the fluorescent bed light for what seemed like the first time all month. Her white hair was neatly brushed and someone had tied it with a fanciful green bow. Her parchment skin folded in fine wrinkles over her tranquil, sleeping face. There was not a trace of agony or stress. Dora's left arm lay open on the bed, atop the neatly tucked white sheet.

There were the numbers.

I hadn't seen them before because I hadn't looked closely. Blue-green numbers, faded with time, but still legible. I had never seen tattooed numbers up close and I wasn't prepared for the reflexive chill that they would cause. Haltingly, I placed my index finger on the numbers. I had never before touched tattooed numbers, and I feared—I don't know what I feared; the numbers were simply frightening to touch.

I rubbed my fingers over her skin tentatively, and the silkiness of this soft side of her arm—the part that had remained free from a lifetime of sun damage—calmed me. The numbers, of course, did not smudge or disappear with my rubbing, despite my irrational thought that they might. I let out the breath that had been caught inside me and leaned in closer. Her fragrance—a combination of baby powder, Betadine, and the vague sourness of the sick—enveloped me and froze me in that moment.

I was touching Dora's skin, the same skin that had been wrenched by a Nazi soldier, stabbed by a metal plate of tattoo needles, and then abraded with blue ink rubbed into the wounds. My fingers could almost feel the shivers and gooseflesh that must have rippled through the supple skin of a teenage girl, one hand stiffened in a soldier's clench, the other gripping the hand of her little sister.

More than a half century later, I was standing in the same position and handling the very same flesh as that Nazi. I shuddered to think of the connection that my fingers were making, that I could have a link with that German soldier whose name would never be known but whose features and touch, I imagined, were seared into Dora's now-quiescent mind. I was grateful that between then and now there had at least been decades of loving touch from a devoted sister and a husband—sixty years of caresses to mitigate, somewhat, the vicious touch that had assaulted the tender underbelly of her arm and branded it with those numbers.

And now I was part of that chain of touch.

The next morning, as I girded myself for battle with the bureaucracy to get my patient transferred back to her nursing home despite the fluctuations of mercury, the intern came up to tell me that Mrs. Millstein had died at 8:20 P.M. the previous night. 8:20 P.M.: thirty minutes after I had left her bedside. I stared at my fingers, rubbing the pads, suddenly entranced by the whorls and creases. Of all the thousands of fingers that had touched Dora in her eighty years of life, from the first that brought her into this world as a fragile infant through the many that had touched her with either violence or affection, could mine have been the last? These calloused bits of skin that I scrub daily and unthinkingly with desiccating antimicrobial soap, that I sheathe and unsheathe with airless latex gloves, that casually grasp my ever-crumpling list of patients may have been the last in this particular chain.

Many industries have been automated, and medicine is no exception. I can't deny the increased efficiency provided by computerized lab results, telemetry monitoring, and wireless e-mail. But no matter how much our field is pushed to streamline and to maximize efficiency, there is an asymptotic limit. In the end, medicine will always be about one patient and one physician together in one room, connecting through the most basic of communication systems: touch. In an age of breathless innovation, this is almost antediluvian. But medicine simply cannot be automated beyond this point.

Every so often, when the chaos of clinic and ward life becomes overwhelming, I dump my computerized list of patients, the review article I've been reading, my Palm Pilot, my triplicate prescription pad, and whatever else I happen to be carrying onto the nearest table. I place my hands flat on the surface, absorbing its comforting smoothness, then spread my fingers and contemplate their outlines. These—more than our stethoscopes, more than our textbooks, more than our clinical practice guidelines—are our most fundamental diagnostic and therapeutic tools. I realize that I am grateful for the inefficiencies of medicine and for their steadfast ineradicability.

And then I gather up my other tools, sigh, and move on.

Acknowledgments

People often ask how I manage to balance doctoring, writing, editing, and raising a family with two small children and one exuberant black lab mutt. The answer is that I do not do it all, and I certainly don't do any of it alone. Each of these activities represents an intricate patchwork of people and relationships. While I do see patients alone in my clinic office, I also work with a brilliant and dedicated group of physicians at Bellevue whose intellectual curiosity and devotion to patient care make this city hospital one of the finest environments in which to work. Their support—along with that of the Department of Medicine at NYU—of my oddball academic career makes it possible to combine writing with clinical medicine.

Writing, at least actually putting words on the page, is admittedly a solitary endeavor (well, Juliet the dog is usually present during those long, lonely days, nosing my hand on the keyboard, inserting an untold number of typos). But after the initial draft, writing is a more communal experience, with the pieces being shaped by a number of hands. Members of my writing group— Thomas Estler, Sandeep Jauhar, Bara Swain, and Sue Scheid—have all offered suggestions that have opened my eyes to new possibilities. The editors at other magazines in which many of these essays have appeared have also helped shape the writing. Debbie Malina and the editorial staff of the *New England Journal of Medicine* have been particularly supportive. It was a steamy August afternoon, and my children were racing up and down the halls of the *NEJM* offices, when I met with the editors and they proposed the idea of publishing something more "literary" in their august, but admittedly somewhat dry, pages. *NEJM*'s decision to publish "Tools of the Trade" provided part of the impetus for this book.

Another part of the development of this book was the involvement of my patients. Unlike those in my first book, some of the essays here were written in real time. For the first time I was able to discuss the writing with my patients. One patient, "Mr. Karlin," read the manuscript of his chapter and contributed voluminous comments. Our discussions enlightened both of us to many of the finer points of both writing and doctoring. His trust and his blessings will not be forgotten.

And at the end of the line (or really at the beginning) is Helene Atwan, my editor at Beacon Press. Her mild-mannered but insistent coaxing overcame my conviction that I couldn't possibly find time for a second book. "It will only hurt a little bit," she said, as she gently bludgeoned entire sections that didn't work. But it was her ongoing optimism that kept it going, along with the enthusiastic support of all the staff at Beacon.

Editing, solitary in the part where one is reading and thinking about another writer's work, is also a group effort. The support and teamwork of the editorial staff of the *Bellevue Literary Review* makes it possible to keep editing an active and viable part of my life.

Raising a family is, by definition, a group effort. I couldn't have found a better partner in this venture than Benjy Akman. He is an incredible father and husband, not to mention a bang-up computer programmer who's pulled me out of more Microsoft pickles than I care to recall. He's also edited everything I've written and has been an uncompromising supporter of my work. Naava and Noah have provided the spice in our lives: the love, the delight, the sleeplessness. In their youthful exuberance they care equally little about editorial deadlines, departmental politics, patient-care responsibilities, and parental sleep. As long as there's adequate peanut butter and cream cheese available, along with crayons and our dog, Juliet, life is good. Thankfully, their effervescent insouciance is occasionally contagious. They remind me not to take any of this too seriously and are endlessly forgiving of my shortcomings.

It is within these intertwining groups that I "do" all these things in my life. My gratitude extends to a chaotic web of interconnected friends, family, canines, colleagues, editors, writers, mentors, doctors, patients, takeout restaurants, delivery people, UPS workers, housecleaners, babysitters, dog walkers, and the sum total of their support. I wouldn't boast this as the most efficient way to write a book, but it certainly isn't dull, and it never gets lonely.

CREDITS

Some of the essays in this book were originally published elsewhere:

Both *Best American Science Writing 2003* and *Tikkun* published "Common Ground"

New England Journal of Medicine published "Torment" and "Tools of the Trade"

The Missouri Review published "Living Will"

JAMA published a portion of "SAT" as "Autopsy Room"

National Public Radio also ran a version of "SAT"

The Annals of Internal Medicine published "Acne"

Rio Grande Review published "Missing the Final Act"

Science & Spirit published "Incidental Findings"

Terminus published "In Her Own Key"